The
McDonald's
Diet

The McDonald's Diet
© 2010 by Mark Austin

ISBN-13: 978-1-4538515-5-5
ISBN-10: 1-4538515-5-0

Find us on the worldwide web at www.austinfitness.ch

Book Design • Leigh Anne Ference-Kaemmer • *www.laferencekaemmer.com*

Photography on Cover and pages vi, 93, 155 • ©Rafa Irusta • Dreamstime.com

Interior Photography • Lisa Trocchi • *www.lisa4photography.com*

The
McDonald's
Diet

How I lost 14 pounds in 30 days
eating nothing but McDonald's

MARK AUSTIN

to the loving memory of Reg Park, my friend and mentor

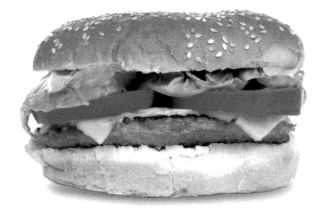

Table of Contents

Introduction

I have been helping people lose weight for the last 27 years now. Clients that I have directly trained in only the last 3 years have lost a combined weight of several tons. Anyone serious about losing weight should keep an eating diary. I look at these diaries between 10 and 20 times a day, every day of my life and I have heard all the excuses:

"We were in a restaurant and there was nothing else to eat"

"We were invited out and I had to eat everything so as not to offend the host"

"It was someone's birthday/wedding/anniversary and we had to celebrate"

"It was Christmas/Easter/Ramadan/Purim and it is traditional to eat that"

"That was all that is available at our company canteen"

"Someone especially baked that for me so I had to eat it"

More than 66% of all Americans are considered to be overweight. That is 2 out of every 3 people. The fast food industry, and particularly McDonald's is often blamed for this.

On the other side of the spectrum, Whole Foods Market is the world's largest retailer of natural and organic foods, and is considered the bastion of good health. Just walking into the Whole Foods Market makes one feel sanctimonious and healthy. McDonald's equals fat and unhealthy, Whole Foods Market equals fit and healthy.

But is this really so ?

I recently walked down the isles of a Whole Foods Market and saw many shelves laden with cakes, cookies, potato crisps, chocolates, white bread etc. Sure they may be natural and organic, but anyone filling their shopping carts with these items is on the fast road to obesity.

So if you can get fat eating food from Whole Foods Market, can you lose weight eating at McDonald's ? As it turns out, you can. I went a full month eating nothing but McDonald's and lost a whole 14 pounds doing so. Fourteen pounds in one month is good on any diet, especially since I was not particularly overweight to start with.

This book documents my journey to discover that the only thing to blame for being overweight is the small choices people make on a daily basis.

What portion size you choose, which dressing, dessert or no dessert, going back for seconds, all of these have a massive bearing on whether you lose or gain weight.

Whether staying in a hotel, visiting a foreign country, partaking in a business lunch, celebrating an occasion or dining at McDonald's, you always have choices. And if your choices in food items are for some reason limited, you always have choices in quantities.

So what may sound like an oxymoron, let's take a look at the McDonald's Weight Loss Plan.

Disclaimer and Caution

This book was written without the author having any affiliation or communication with the McDonald's Corporation of any nature.

All the information presented in this book is for entertainment, educational and resource purposes only. It is NOT a substitute for any advice given to you by your physician or health care provider. Always consult your physician or health care provider before beginning any nutrition or exercise program. Use of the information contained in this book is at the sole choice and risk of the reader.

We are NOT LIABLE for any injury, losses or damages which may occur through your use of any information or products which you obtain through reading this book.

Always warm up thoroughly before training.

Any activity which loads, bends or twists your spine in any way should be avoided for the first hour after rising. This is because during sleep the spine fills with a fluid for purposes of nourishment, making it very sensitive for that first hour.[1]

My first stop was a visit to Dr. Roland Dillinger, a medical doctor practicing in Niederweningen, a town 15 miles north of Zurich, Switzerland.

Dr. Dillinger examined me thoroughly, took blood to test my cholesterol and liver function, X-rayed my chest and weighed me.

He found me to be in excellent health, except when he got my liver function results back they were rather high.

I would return to him exactly 30 days later for the same examination. Until then the only solid foods I would eat would all be purchased from McDonald's.

I was going to make every day a McDonald's day.

The Results

	Before	After
Body Weight	166 pounds	152 pounds
Body Fat	16%	9%
Cholesterol		
Total	234	147
LDL	142	80
Liver Function		
AST (GOT)	94.3	39.8
ALT (GPT)	443	46.8

Notes:

>> *I lost 14 pounds in 30 days.*

>> *My body fat went from 16%, which is considered normal, to 9%, which is considered to be that of an athlete[1]*

>> *My total cholesterol went from 234 which is considered to be too high to 147 which is very good. [2]*

>> *My LDL (the bad cholesterol) went from 142 which is borderline high down to 80 which is optimal. [3]*

AST and ALT are enzymes made in the liver. High levels of these enzymes in the bloodstream are indicative of problems with the liver. The normal ranges are under 43 IU/L and under 60 IU/L respectively.[4]

>> *My AST levels were nearly double the healthy level and my ALT levels were more than 7 times higher before the diet. Both were within the healthy range after the diet.*

>> *I do not drink alcohol or take any medications so the reason for the high levels was probably excessive protein and fat intake.*

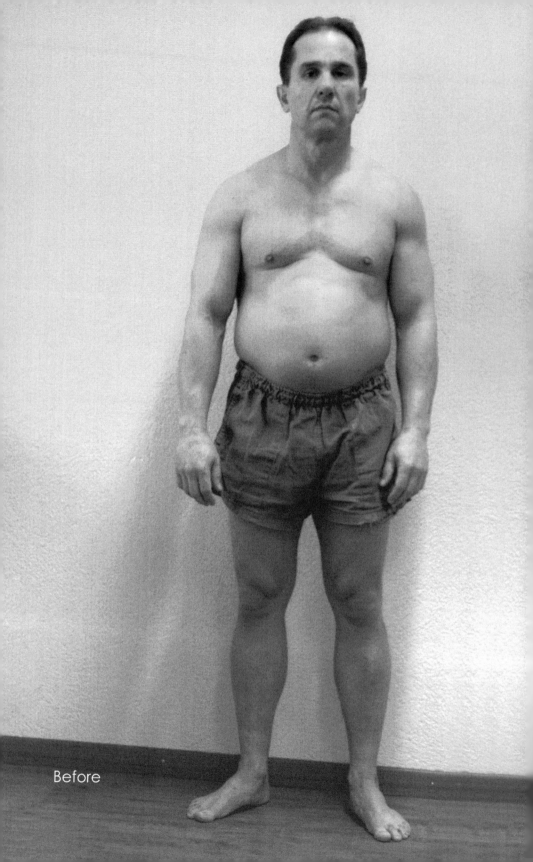

Before

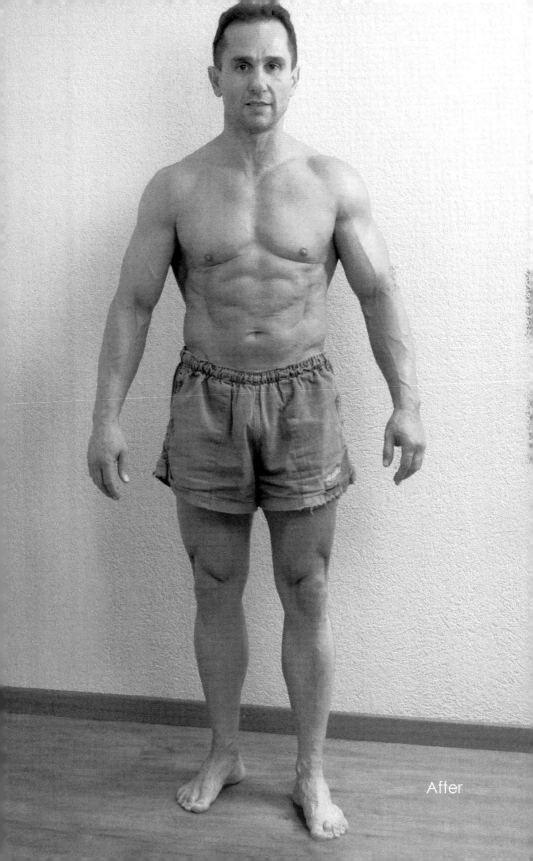
After

Supplementation

Regardless of what eating plan you follow it is always sensible to supplement your diet with certain nutrients that your solid food intake alone is unlikely to provide.

A Multivitamin

A good daily multivitamin and Mineral is essential to ensure against any gaps in your nutrition which may compromise your health and well-being. Few people eat the recommended 5 - 9 portions of fruit and vegetables **every single day.**[1] A lot of people don't even get that in a week. And for those who do, with modern farming practices (read squeeze everything out of the earth as cheaply as possible), even if you do, produce does not have the nutritional value it once did.

Ask your pharmacist or health care provider to recommend a good one for you, as grabbing the first one you see on the supermarket shelf is not a good idea.

Fish Oil

Fish Oil has been proven to protect against heart diseases[2], reduce fatty deposits in arteries, reduce feelings of depression and anxiety[3], reduce the risk of all forms of cancer, help alleviate the symptoms of arthritis[4], tendonitis and all other inflammatory conditions. It is also very important for effective weight loss[5]. There are so many well documented benefits to taking fish oil that anyone who does not eat a large portion of fatty fish every day should absolutely supplement with fish oil. Again ask your pharmacist to recommend a brand and dosage appropriate for you.

Protein

Anyone engaging in vigorous exercise should consume about ½ to 1 gram of protein for every pound of body weight per day.[6] This should be spread across 4 to 5 "feeds" throughout the day. I use the word "feeds" as opposed to "meals" because a protein shake or bar may be more convenient at certain times of the day. Protein bars either taste disgusting or they are loaded with carbohydrates, so a protein drink is usually better. **Whey Protein Concentrate** or **Whey Protein Isolate** are good choices, and make sure they are not sweetened with Aspartame or its derivatives.

Other Supplements

There are literally thousands of other supplements out there. Some of them are beneficial and some of them have absolutely no benefit. Unless you have been advised otherwise by your health care provider, stick to the above 3 and you should be good. Most supplements claiming to drastically accelerate your weight loss have very little use and you will lose more weight on your wallet than on your waist by taking them.

The Diet

As you probably already assumed, the McDonald's Salads formed a very big part of my diet. Every thing you have ever heard about weight loss, every article you have ever read and every scientific study that has ever been done can be summarized in these two points :

In order to lose body fat the number of calories you expend each day must exceed the number of calories you consume, and you must manage your insulin levels.

Let's look at this in more detail.

1) To reduce the number of calories you consume you must

- Eat less calorie dense foods
- Eat more fiber and water rich foods
- Reduce the quantity of food

2) To increase the number of calories you expend you must

- Do more physical "work"
- Increase the rate at which your body burns calories at rest (your Basal Metabolic Rate or BMR)

3) To manage your insulin levels you must

- Avoid foods with a high Glycemic Index
- Eat 4 to 5 smaller meals per day, rather than 2 or 3 larger ones
- Exercise more, and especially high intensity exercise like that described in the chapters on Strength Training and Metabolic Disturbance

Calorie Dense Foods include

Sugary Foods and Drinks: smoothies, fruit juices, sodas, alcohol, biscuits, cakes, doughnuts, candies, breakfast cereals and cereal bars, preserves, most types of dessert, dates

Starches: foods containing wheat, meal, flour or corn (bread, pasta, pizza base etc), oatmeal, Quinoa, potatoes, yams, maize, rice, beans (other than green beans)

High Fat Foods: butter, margarine, all types of edible oil, coconut and coconut milk, batter, ice cream, most cheeses, doughnuts, potato chips, fatty cuts of meat, most processed meats like sausages, salami and pepperoni, chicken skin and chicken wings, duck, mayonnaise, most sauces and dressings, all nuts and nut spreads, chocolate

Fiber and Water Rich Foods include

Most Vegetables: artichoke, asparagus, beet, broccoli, Brussels sprouts, cabbage, cauliflower, celery, chard, chicory, cucumber, eggplant, kale, kohlrabi, leek, mushrooms, onions, radish, rhubarb, spinach, zucchini

Most Salad Ingredients: alfalfa sprouts, celery, lettuce (all types), onions, tomatoes, watercress

Reducing the quantity of food

This may not be as hard as it sounds. We eat for enjoyment, for comfort, for entertainment, for nourishment and to satisfy hunger.

If you were to eat portions half the size of what you currently eat, but chew twice as long as you do at the moment, you would gain all the benefits that you currently gain by eating the way you do. But you would also halve your calorie intake.

Enjoyment: Food actually tastes much better if you chew it a lot more. Certain enzymes are released in your mouth which start the digestive process while you are chewing, and these enzymes improve the taste of the food.

Comfort: The comfort you gain from eating food is related to the enjoyment and the feeling satisfied. As stated above these qualities are enhanced with more chewing.

Entertainment is doing something to pass the time which is enjoyable. Chewing twice as much makes it more enjoyable and takes just as long as eating double the portion size faster.

Nourishment: Chewing longer improves the digestion of your food and therefore is more nourishing. Half way into most meals you have enough food to satisfy your need for nourishment. The rest goes straight to your hips or belly.

Satisfaction: The systems our body use to let us know that we have had enough to eat have about a fifteen minute delay. This means that we only know that we have had enough fifteen minutes after we actually have had enough. If you eat fast you can take in 300 to 500 calories in that fifteen minutes. Chewing longer will allow you to feel full before you have over-eaten.

Physical Work is done every time you move any part of your body, whether it is to walk, swim, stand up, or to lift or move some object. Physical work is calculated by considering the force it takes to move an object (including your own body) and the distance the object is moved. So if you want to increase the amount of physical work done we can increase the resistance (the weight load by for example lifting heavier weights when exercising) or do more repetitions with the same resistance (do it for longer), or increase both.

Basal Metabolic Rate is influenced by a number of things, but we will only consider the factors which you can positively influence. These include muscle mass, the thermogenic affect of food and body fat pecentage.

Muscle needs calories just to sustain itself, even at rest. So the more muscle you have, the more calories you burn at rest. This is a major reason why it gets harder to lose weight as we age. Without intervention we lose muscle mass every year after the age of 25[1].

This is also a major reason for the yo-yo effect of dieting. If you lose weight with diet alone, a lot of that weight (25 - 50%) is muscle[2]. When you start eating normally again, your body needs far fewer calories to sustain itself, and so you rapidly gain the weight back. But most of the weight you gain back is fat. The result of years of up and down dieting is a metabolism that is so slow that the number of calories needed just to maintain your weight is less than the number of calories needed to nourish the body.

The only way to prevent this is to do strength training while you limit your calorie intake.

Women need not fear that building muscle will make them look masculine. Without taking male hormones you will not be able to build muscles like a man even if you wanted to. The more muscle you build, the faster you lose fat and the easier it is to maintain your desired weight once you have reached it. Muscle also gives your body an attactive shape and a toned appearance. *Everyone needs more muscle!*

The Thermogenic Effect of Food refers to how the body burns calories to digest food. Almost ⅓ of the calories in protein are used to digest that protein. Carbohydrates use only 7% of the calories to digest them, and fats 3%. So if you eat 100 calories each of protein, carbohydrates and fat, only about 70 of the protein calories will remain after they are digested, 93 of the carbohydrates, and 97 of the fat calories will be available to make you fat.[3]

Managing Insulin Levels

Insulin is one of the most anabolic of all hormones. This means it causes growth. Under most circumstances this is bad because that growth is in the form of fat. But directly after heavy strength training the growth is muscle. So the goal is to avoid surges in our insulin levels most of the time, except around our strength workouts. More about this later.

High Glycemic Index foods cause a surge in insulin levels. The Glycemic Index (GI) is a scale which shows the effect that different foods have on our sugar levels and therefore our insulin levels. Foods with the highest GI spike insulin levels the most. The more carbohydrates there are in the food, the higher the GI. So all the foods listed above as Sugary Foods and Starches should be avoided.

Eating several small meals a day also helps to ensure a constant insulin level. If there are any carbohydrates in your food at all, there will be some rise in insulin. So if you eat the same number of carbohydrates but spread over more meals, each individual rise will be less. Four or five meals a day takes advantage of this concept without being impractical.

Strength Training and Metabolic Disturbance Training reduce the effect of insulin spikes for two reasons. Firstly insulin output goes down and secondly insulin is absorbed more rapidly during exercise.

When you can and should eat lots of Carbohydrates

Peri Workout Nutrition (Nutrition just before, during and right after)

Intense exercise initially causes a break down of muscle, which then leads to rebuilding of new muscle. An insulin spike around the time of your workout will reduce the muscle break down and increase the rebuilding. Some estimates say that the results of your workouts will be increased by as much as 30% with proper Peri Workout Nutrition.[4]

In short, it is good to have an insulin spike at this time, which means that you should eat a carbohydrate rich meal. The meal should also contain a lot of protein to help build the muscle, but no fat, as this slows digestion, which decreases the insulin spike.

So straight after all my Strength Training workouts I would eat either a Mc Chicken Burger or a chicken wrap without sauces, as they are both high in protein and carbohydrate. Any of the Hamburger choices would also be fine.

The advantages of eating a meal high in carbohydrates and protein are

- **decreases muscle breakdown**

- **increases muscle building**

- **gives you something to look forward to while you are dieting**

- **stops your body from evoking the starvation response which makes it harder to lose weight**[5]

Drinks

I pretty much stuck to drinking water right the way through the diet. I would rather eat my calorie allowance than waste it on drinks. Drink as much water as you can comfortably tolerate whether it be warm, hot, iced, still, sparking, filtered, tap, with a dash of lemon juice (but not a dash of whiskey) etc.

Exercise

No weight loss plan, no health plan, no success plan, no happiness plan would ever be complete without physical exercise playing a substantial role.

Physical Exercise

- **Improves your mood**
- **Makes you look and feel younger and better**
- **Combats chronic diseases**
- **Helps you to lose weight**
- **Boosts your energy levels**
- **Reduces stress**
- **Promotes better sleep**
- **Improves your sex life**

The list goes on and on.

This is my favorite quote regarding exercise, and it comes from one of the world's leading authorities:

"While Chronological age is invariable, physiological age has a variable of 30 years. You can have the external appearance and internal system of someone 15 years older, or 15 years younger than you are. The right kind of exercise buys us years."[1]

Three types of exercise are required to give you optimum results, namely **Strength Training** which allows you to move with greater force. **Cardiovascular Training** which allows you to move for longer periods of time and the third type includes **Flexibility, Mobility and other activities** to improve the quality of your movements.

Strength Training:

- **helps you to maintain muscle mass while you lose weight so that the weight you lose is fat, not muscle**

- **builds muscle which makes your body stronger and more toned**

- **increases your Basal Metabolic Rate (BMR), which is the rate at which your body burns calories while at rest. If your BMR is higher you literally burn more calories while you are sitting still or even asleep**

- **boosts your levels of growth hormone which makes you leaner, stronger and look younger in every way[2]**

The strength program I followed is called an upper body / lower body split, which means I trained my upper body the one workout (workout A) and my lower body the next (workout B)

I trained 3 times per week: For most people training on Monday, Wednesday and Friday would work best. Because of my work schedule, however, I trained on Sunday, Tuesday and Thursday. One week you would do workout A twice, and B once. The next week it would be B twice and A once.

So 2 weeks would look like this:

Monday	workout A
Tuesday	no strength training
Wednesday	workout B
Thursday	no strength training
Friday	workout A
Saturday	no strength training
Sunday	no strength training
Monday	workout B
Tuesday	no strength training
Wednesday	workout A
Thursday	no strength training
Friday	workout B
Saturday	no strength training
Sunday	no strength training

In the following chapter you will find all the strength training exercises I did, with photos and a brief description or tips where required.

In most cases there is one photo of two people demonstrating each exercise. The one person will be in the start / finish position from the front, and the other person will be in the midway position from the side.

Because so many people grasp a movement better when they actually see it being performed I also made a video of each exercise. If you go to my website at *www.austinfitness.ch* and click The McDonald's Diet and then on the Exercise Videos tab you will find a list of all the exercises in this book in the order in which they appear.

Wherever you see this symbol in this book 📹 there is a video of it.

Any term that you read in the book that is followed by a (G) is defined more fully in the Glossary at the end.

Progressions and Regressions

For progress to be made with any physical exercise it is important that it is possible to make the exercise more challenging as you adapt to the exercise.

Most exercises can be made more challenging simply by increasing the number of repetitions (G). Different "Rep Ranges" (G) have different results however, so doing more and more repetitions will not always give the benefit we are looking for.

Any exercise which involves lifting an external load (for example a dumbbell (G) or a barbell (G) or a kettlebell (G) or any exercise machine) can be made more challenging by increasing the weight.

If an exercise involves only your body weight for resistance (G), then progressions become a little more complicated.

A more difficult version of an exercise is called a Progression.

Regressions are the opposite of Progressions and involve making an exercise easier.

If you follow the program I did, you would only move on to the progression of a specific exercise when you are able to perform the correct number of repetitions in good exercise form (G). If you are unable to perform the basic exercise in good form, then start with the regression.

Alternating Sets

If an exercise called for multiple sets (G) to be performed, then I would group 2 or 3 exercises together. So instead of doing a set of one exercise and then sitting around to recover before I started the second set, I would alternate between 2 or 3 different exercises, taking just a short rest between each. This gives the individual muscles a longer time to recover between sets but cuts right down on the total rest time. Because the muscles have more time to recover, you will be able to lift heavier weights, and because the total rest time is much shorter, you will be able to get a lot more done in a shorter time, i.e. your training intensity will be much higher.

To indicate alternating sets I number them on my workout 1a, 1b, 2a, 2b, 2c etc. which would mean that I would alternate between exercises 1a and 1b until all the sets for those two exercises were complete and then I would alternate between 2a, 2b and 2c.

```
***********************************

        MCDONALD'S Restaurant
        NIEDERHASLISTRASSE 7
        8157 DIELSDORF
        Tel 044 854 06 09
        Hern Beat Zobrist


***********************************


        Vielen Dank für Ihren Besuch
        McDonald's wünscht Ihnen einen
             excellenten Appetit


***********************************

              QUITTUNG

No TVA: MWST NR 265 914#ORD 87
05/05/2010 15:30:10
ANZ PROD
    5 CA-GRILLED
    5 FRUIT BAG
    5 BALSAMICO

    Eat-In Total
    CHF
    Change

    TAX A ( 7,60%)        59.

    ***         Oeffnungsz
    Montag - Donnerstag
    Freitag und Samstag
    Sonntag
    =======================
```

```
***********************************

            MCDONALD'S Restaurant
            NIEDERHASLISTRASSE 7
            8157 DIELSDORF
            Tel 044 854 06 09
            Hern Beat Zobrist


***********************************


        Vielen Dank für Ihren Besuch
        McDonald's wünscht Ihnen einen
             excellenten Appetit

***********************************


              QUITTUNG

No TVA: MWST NR 265 914#ORD 91 -REG 3-
21/04/2010 15:38:00
ANZ PROD
    1 SMAL VALSER                TOTAL
    4 CA-GRILLED                  3.50
    1 SMAL SALAT                 39.60
    1 6-NUGGETS                   3.00
    6 FRUIT BAG                   5.90
    4 BALSAMICO                  12.00
    1 BARBECUE SAUCE              0.00

    Take-Out Total                0.00
    CHF                          64.00
    Change                      214.00
                                150.00
    TAX B ( 2.40%)     64.00 =
                                  1.50
    ***        Oeffnungszeiten         ***
    Montag - Donnerstag :  08h30 - 23h30
    Freitag und Samstag :  08h30 - 01h00
    Sonntag             :  10h30 - 23h30
    =================================
```

The Exercises

Prone Plank

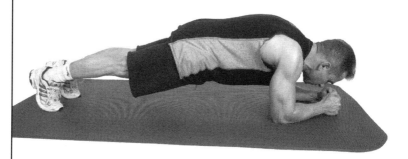

Main muscles: Core including abdominals (stomach muscles)

1. Clench your butt muscles and hold your stomach muscles tight as though you were bracing against a punch to the stomach.

2. Do not allow your lower back to sag.

3. Hold this position for the required number of seconds.

4. Because this is a static exercise, there is no video.

Regression: **Prone Plank on Knees**

If you cannot hold the Prone Plank for 10 seconds or more then do it with your knees on the floor. Your thighs and back should be in a straight line.

like this   not this

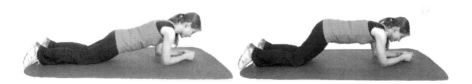

Once you can hold the Prone Plank on Knees for 40 seconds or more, try the Prone Plank again.

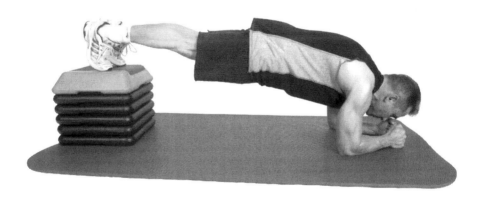

Progression: **Incline Prone Plank**

When you can hold the prone Plank for 60 seconds then do it with your feet raised.

Side Plank

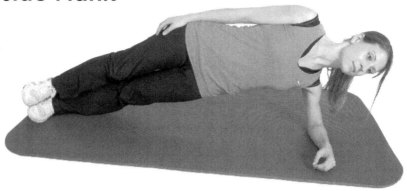

**Main muscles: Core including obliques ("love-handles"),
quadratus lumborum**

1. Do not allow your hips to sag down.

2. Make sure that your body is straight, i.e. push your hips slightly
   forward and don't allow your hips to rotate backwards.

Regression: **Side Plank on Knees**

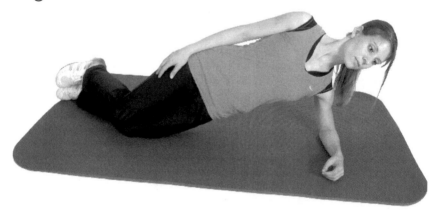

Progression: **Side Plank with Weight**

Rest a dumbbell on your top thigh (No Photo)

🎥 Bird Dog

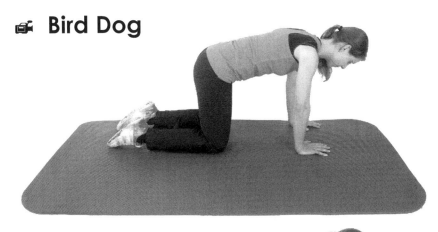

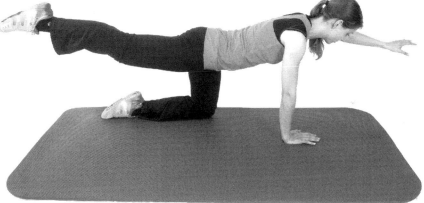

Main muscle: Lower back
Other muscles: Buttocks, back of thighs, abdominals

1. Start on all fours with your shoulders directly above your hands and your hips directly above your knees.

2. Keeping your stomach muscles tight raise opposite arm and leg and hold for 2 seconds

3. Your pelvis must not rotate.

Progression: **Bird Dog with Weight**

Put ankle weights around your ankles and hold a dumbbell in your hand

🎥 Mc Gill Crunch

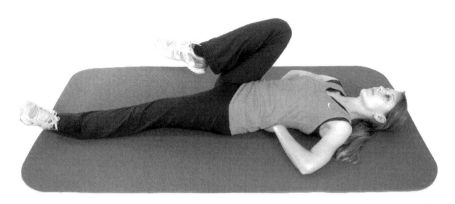

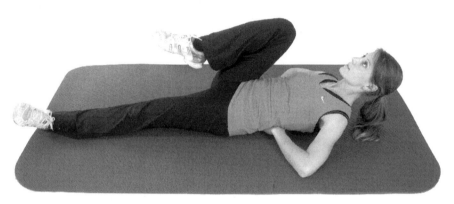

Main muscle: Abdominals

1. Put your hands under the small of your back to prevent your lower back from flattening.

2. Hold the up position for 3 seconds while tighly flexing your stomach muscles.

3. Be sure not to push down into the floor with your elbows.

🎥 Pallof Press

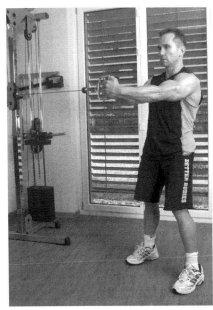 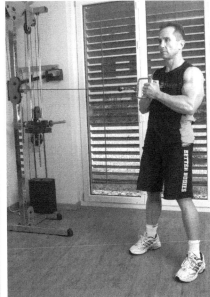

Main muscles: Core stabilizers

1. Brace your core to prevent the weight from rotating your torso.

2. Extend your arms and hold for the required time.

3. When extended your forearms should form a 90° angle with the cable.

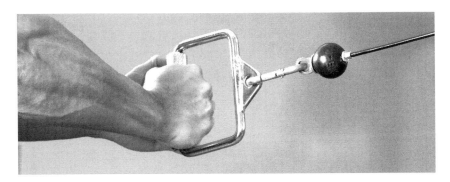

⬛ Ab Wheel Rollouts

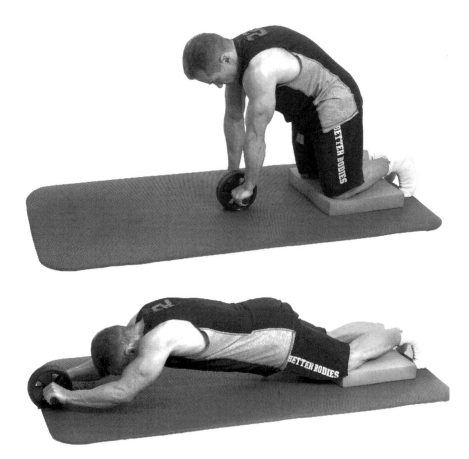

Main muscles: Anterior Core including abdominals
Other muscles: Arms, chest, shoulders, lats

1. Tense your stomach and buttocks muscles and push your hips slightly forward.

2. As you roll forward keep those muscles tight so that your lower back doesn't sag down.

3. If this exercise hurts your back then try the regression.

Regression: 🖭 **Ball rollouts**

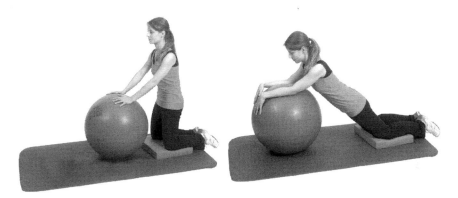

Same instructions as Ab Wheel Rollouts.

If this hurts your back then stick with the Prone Plank and its progressions until your core and back are strong enough to do this without back pain.

📹 45° Back extensions

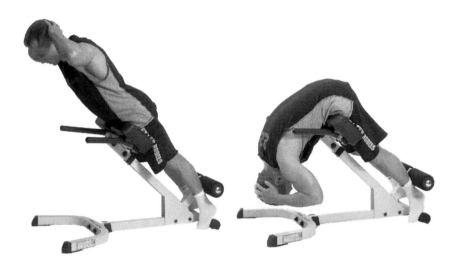

Main muscle: Lower back
Other muscles: Buttocks, back of thighs

1. Raise your torso until your legs and torso are in a straight line. Do NOT go higher than that.

2. Hold at the top position for 3 seconds and lower to the count of 3 seconds.

Some gyms only have flat back extension benches which make the exercise a little more difficult, but the instructions for use are the same.

📹 Reverse Hypers

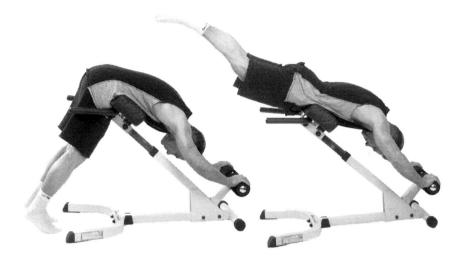

Main muscle: Lower back, buttocks, back of thighs

1. Raise your legs with knees straight until your legs and torso are in a straight line. Do NOT go higher than that.

2. Hold at the top position for 3 seconds and lower to the count of 3 seconds.

Some gyms only have flat back extension benches, but the instructions for use are the same.

The Deadlift

Possibly the most important of all strength exercises. This exercise strengthens more muscles in your body than any other exercise. It builds the most useful strength because in every day life the heaviest weights you have to lift are from the floor to waist height, which is exactly what the deadlift is.

There are many different versions of the deadlift. The following three are the ones I used :

📹 Romanian Deadlift

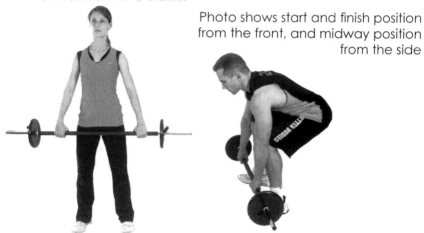

Photo shows start and finish position from the front, and midway position from the side

Main muscles: Lower back, back of thighs, buttocks
Other muscles: Thighs, lats, calves, forearms and grip

1. Lower the bar by pushing your hips back and only slightly bending your knees.

2. The bar should stay close to you at all times and your back must stay straight.

3. Only go as low as you can without rounding your back.

Have somebody check you from the side to make sure you don't round your back.

📷 Sumo Style Romanian Deadlift

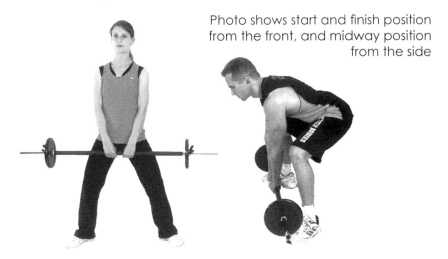

Photo shows start and finish position from the front, and midway position from the side

The same as the Romanian Deadlift, except that your grip is very narrow and your feet are wide and out at 45°.

📷 Snatch Grip Romanian Deadlift

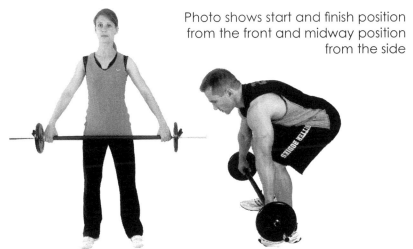

Photo shows start and finish position from the front and midway position from the side

The same as the Romanian Deadlift, except that your grip is very wide.

📷 Body Weight Squat

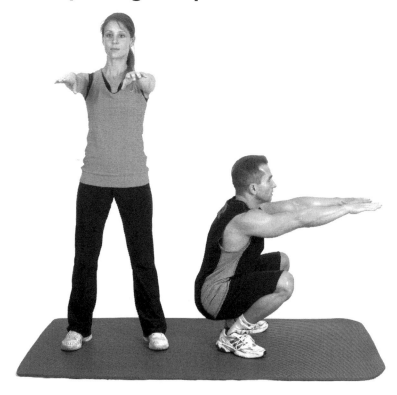

Main muscle: Thighs
Other muscles: Buttocks, back of thighs

1. Keep your back straight and chest up i.e. don't bend forward as you go down.

2. Keep your heels flat on the floor.

3. If you cannot descend without bending forward or lifting your heels then you have mobility issues in your ankles, hips or calves. For now you can correct this by putting a 2 – 3 inch platform under your heels. A piece of wood, weight plates or even a telephone directory will work. This is a short term solution as your mobility issues should be addressed.

Regression: 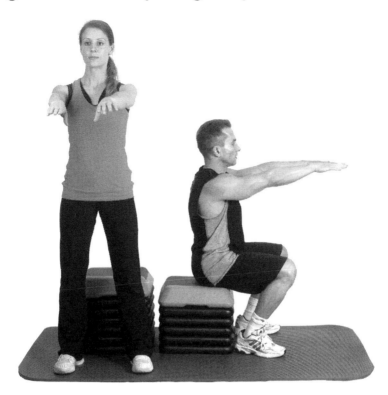 Body Weight Squat to Chair

Main muscle: Thighs
Other muscles: Buttocks, back of thighs

If you are unable to squat down with your own body weight then place a sturdy chair or something similar behind you and squat to that. As you get stronger and more mobile you can use a lower platform to squat to until you can remove it altogether.

⸙ Goblet Squat

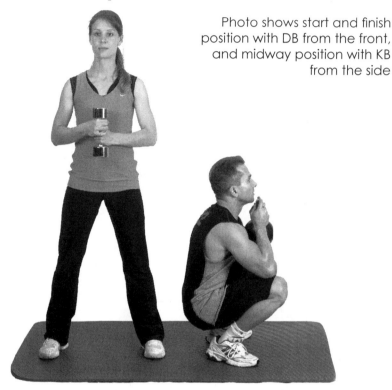

Photo shows start and finish position with DB from the front, and midway position with KB from the side

Resistance is added to the Body Weight Squat by holding a dumbbell or kettlebell at chest height. In addition to training all the muscles the Body Weight Squat trains, this increases the training effect on your core as well as your upper body.

📷 Barbell Front Squat

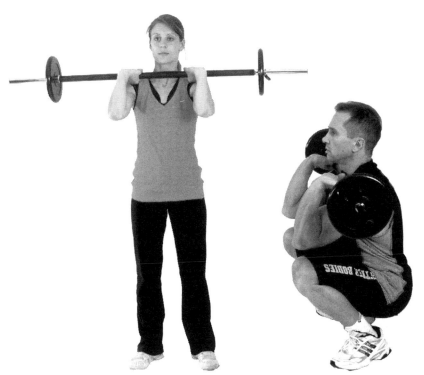

Resistance is added to the Body Weight Squat by holding a barbell across the front of your shoulders. This has the same additional benefits as the Goblet Squat.

📹 Dumbbell Split Squat

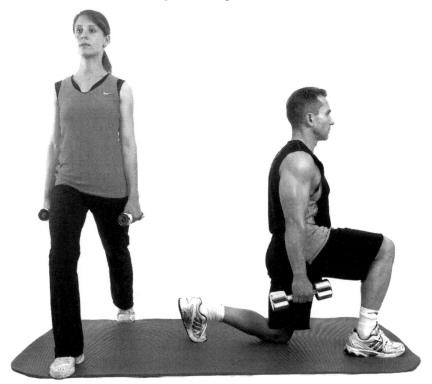

Main muscle: Thighs
Other muscles: Buttocks, back of thighs

1. Start with one foot about 3 feet in front of the other, both knees and feet should always point forward.

2. Keep your back erect, i.e. don't lean forward.

3. Bend your knees so that the knee of the back leg lightly touches the floor and then straighten your knees again to return to the start position.

4. The movement is up and down, rather than forward and back. (Forward and back would be called a static lunge)

📹 Dumbbell or Barbell Forward Lunge

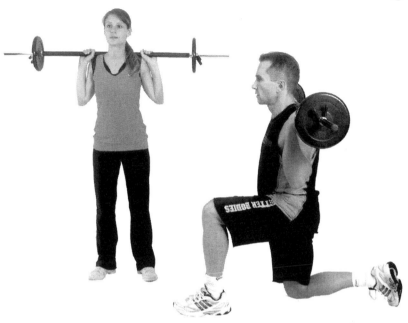

Main muscle: Thighs
Other muscles: Buttocks, back of thighs

1. Start with your feet parallel and close to each other.

2. Take a big step forward and bend your knees so that the knee of your back leg lightly touches the floor.

3. Then push yourself back up to the start position with your front leg and bring your feet together again.

4. Both knees and feet should always point forward.

5. Keep your back erect, i.e. don't lean forward.

Use a barbell only if you have no balance issues. If you do have balance issues then do the exercise holding a pair of dumbbells at your sides.

For greater range of motion you can lunge to a step as shown in the video.

📷 Dumbbell or Barbell Reverse Lunge

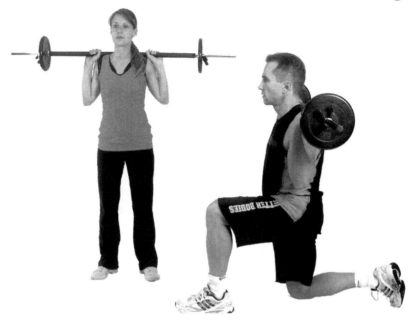

This is the same photo used to illustrate the barbell lunge because the start, finish and midway positions all look the same

Main muscle: Thighs
Other muscles: Buttocks, back of thighs

1. Start with your feet together.

2. Take a big step backward and bend your knees so that the knee of your back leg lightly touches the floor.

3. Then reverse the movement and come back up to the start position using mostly the power from your front leg, rather than pushing up very strongly with your back leg.

4. Both knees and feet should always point forward.

5. Keep your back erect, i.e. don't lean forward.

Use a barbell only if you have no balance issues. If you do have balance issues then do the exercise holding a pair of dumbbells at your sides.

Dumbbell or Barbell Reverse Lunge from a Deficit

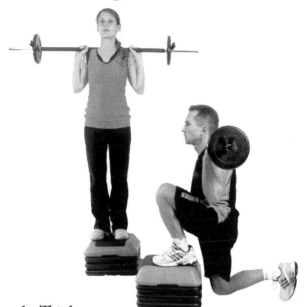

Main muscle: Thighs
Other muscles: Buttocks, back of thighs

1. Start by standing on a step with your feet together.

2. Take a step backward and bend your knees so that the knee of your back leg lightly touches the floor. If you cannot do this then use a lower step.

3. Then reverse the movement and come back up to the start position using mostly the power from your front leg, rather than pushing up very strongly with your back leg.

4. Both knees and feet should always point forward.

5. Keep your back erect, i.e. don't lean forward.

Use a barbell only if you have no balance issues. If you do have balance issues then do the exercise holding a pair of dumbbells at your sides.

⚏ Dumbbell or Barbell Bulgarian Split Squat

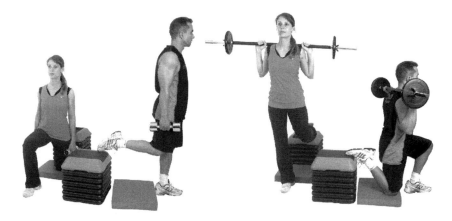

Possibly the hardest exercise I know. They improve hip mobility and flexibility, improve your balance, work your entire lower body and tax your cardiovascular system so you are gasping for air by the end of the set. They are so hard, but they are really worth doing because they do so much.

1. Your back knee should descend to within 2 – 3 inches of the floor.

2. The top of your back foot (shoelace side) should be on the bench.

3. Keep your back erect, i.e. don't lean forward.

4. Use a barbell only if you have no balance issues.

📹 Incline Dumbbell Press

Main muscle: Chest
Secondary muscles: Shoulders, Triceps

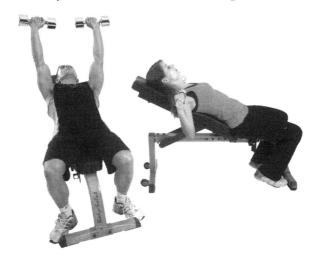

📹 Decline Dumbbell Press

Main muscle: Chest
Secondary muscles: Shoulders, Triceps

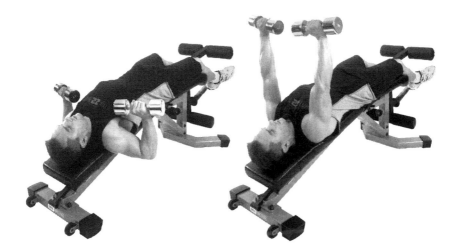

📽 Flat Barbell Press

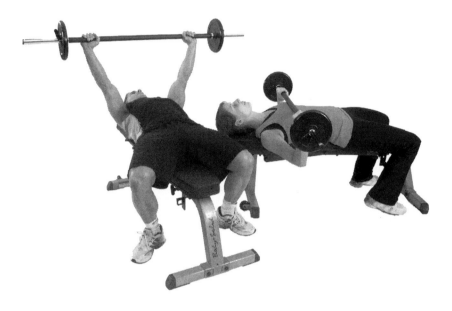

Main muscle: Chest
Secondary muscles: Shoulders, Triceps

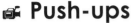 Push-ups

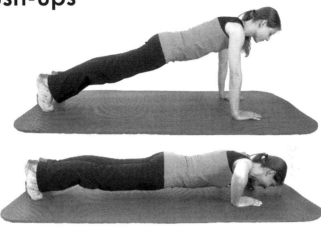

Main muscle: Chest
Secondary muscles: Shoulders, Triceps, Core including Abdominals

1. Your legs, spine and neck should stay in a straight line throughout the exercise.

2. Your chin, chest and pubis should lightly touch the floor at the same time at the bottom of the movement.

Regression: 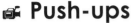 Decline Push-ups

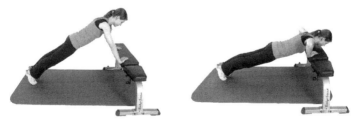

1. Your legs, spine and neck should stay in a straight line throughout.

2. Do not raise your hips.

3. Your chest should lightly touch the bench at the bottom of the movement.

4. The higher your hands are, the easier the exercise is. Placing your hands on the bar of a Smith Machine or Squat Rack allows you

to start with your hands as high as you need to in order to get the required number of repetitions. As you get stronger you can lower the height of the bar. This concept is illustrated in the description of the Horizontal Pull-up on pages 58 & 59.

Progression: 📷 **Push-ups on Stands**

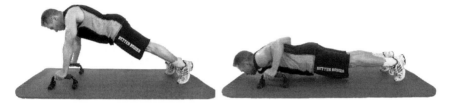

Using push-up stands gives you a greater range of motion

Alternative Progression: 📷 **Incline Push-ups**

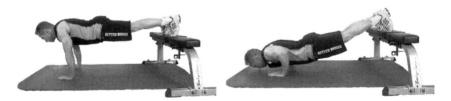

1. Your legs, spine and neck should stay in a straight line throughout.

2. Do not allow your lower back to sag.

Alternative Progression: **Weighted Push-ups**

Wearing a weighted vest allows you to add resistance to the push-up.

In addition any of the push-up progression alternatives can be combined to make it harder. The hardest being Incline Weighted Push-ups on Stands.

▣ Seated Row

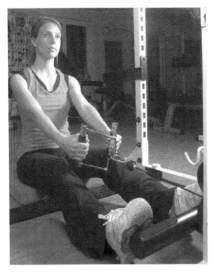 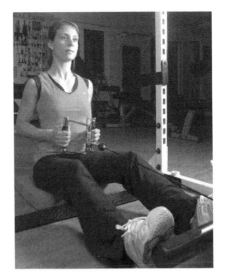

Main muscle: Lats (G)
Secondary muscles: Back of shoulders, biceps, forearms and lower back

1. Keep your torso still and at 90° to the floor.

2. Your back should be slightly arched and your chest sticking out.

3. When the handle touches your stomach squeeze your shoulder blades together and hold that position for 1-2 seconds before returning to the start position.

▣ One Arm Cable Row

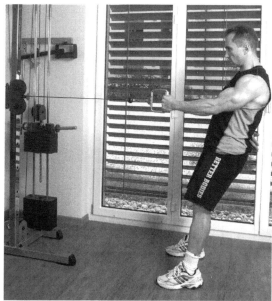

Main and secondary muscles:

Same as seated row plus core stabilizers

Don't rotate your upper body.

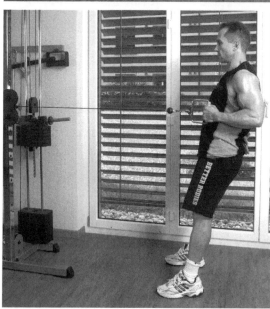

📷 Three Point One Arm Bent Over Dumbbell Row

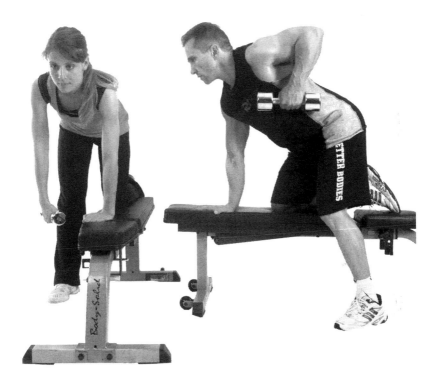

Main and secondary muscles: Same as One arm cable row, but with less core

1. Keep your chest high.

2. Don't rotate your upper body.

📹 Horizontal Pull-up

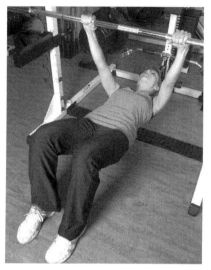 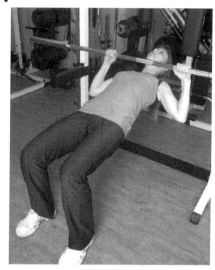

Main and secondary muscles: Same as One Arm Cable Row

1. Your legs, spine and neck should stay in a straight line throughout.

2. No sagging at the hips.

3. The further forward your feet are, the more difficult the exercise is.

Regression: 📷 Set the bar much higher

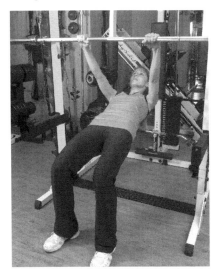 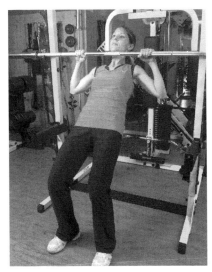

As you get stronger you can lower the bar incrementally.

Progression: 📷 Raise your feet

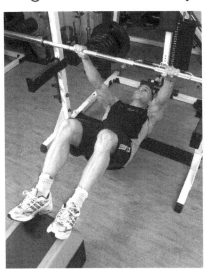 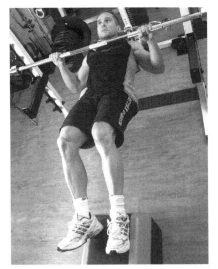

▣ Neutral Grip (G) Pull-downs

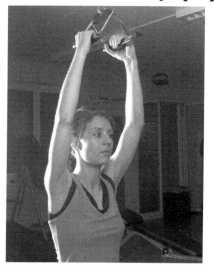 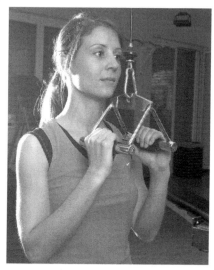

Main muscle: Lats (G)
Secondary muscles: Biceps, forearms and middle back

▣ Pronated Grip (G) Pull-downs

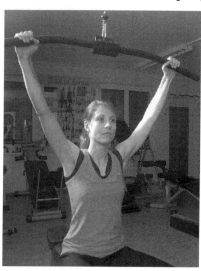

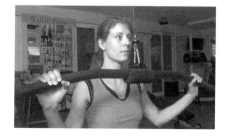

Main muscle: Lats (G)
Secondary muscles:
Biceps, forearms and
middle back

📷 Supinated Grip (G) Pull-downs

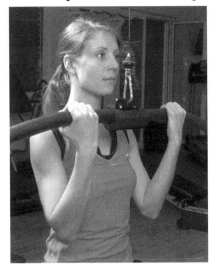 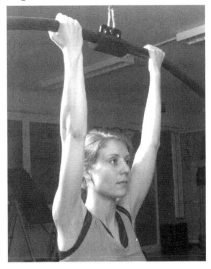

Main muscle: Lats (G)
Secondary muscles: Biceps, forearms and middle back

Progression: ✍ **Pull-ups using the various grips**

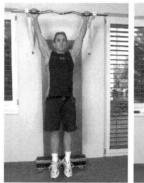 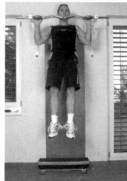

Pronated Grip

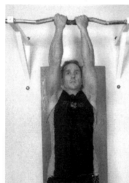 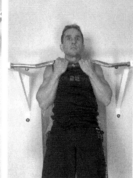

Supinated Grip

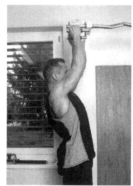 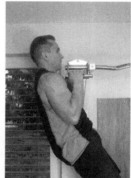

Neutral Grip

Main and secondary muscles :
Same as all the pull-down variations plus massive involvement
of the core stabilizers including the abdominals.

📹 Dumbbell Military Press

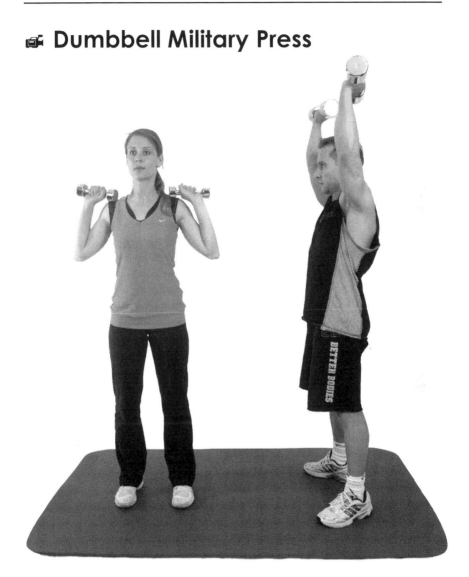

Main muscle: Shoulders
Secondary muscles: Triceps, core stabilizers

Keep your knees slightly bent, buttocks tensed and your abdominals braced (as if expecting a punch in the stomach) throughout the movement.

📹 Neutral Grip Dumbbell Military Press

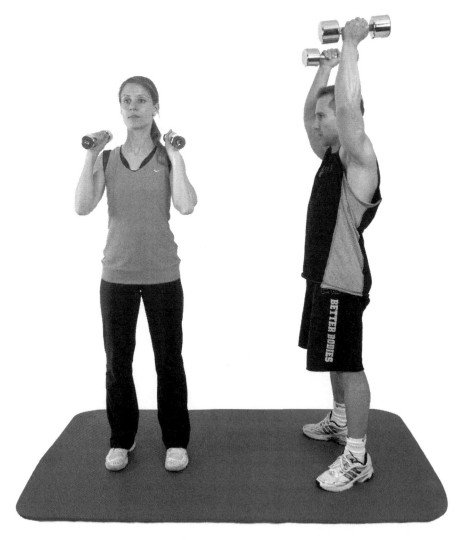

Instructions and muscles worked: Same as Dumbbell Military Press

📷 Alternating Pronating Standing Dumbbell Press

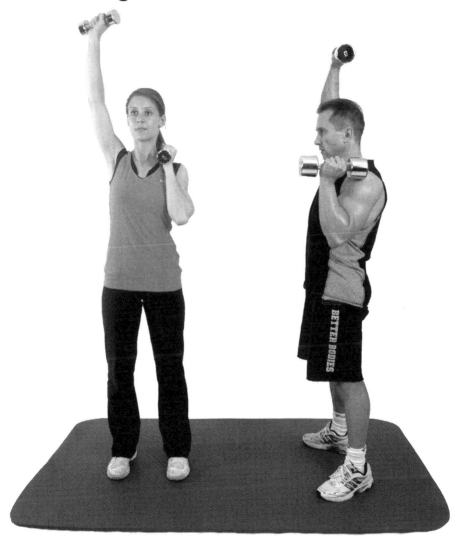

Main and secondary muscles: Same as Dumbbell Military Press

1. As your press the dumbbell up rotate your hand so that your palm faces forward.

2. Rotate it back as you lower

⏵ Seated Arnold Press

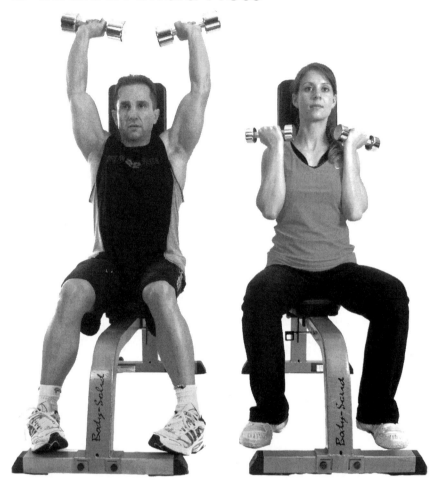

Main muscle: Shoulders
Secondary muscles: Triceps

Named after the Governator, this is one of his favorite shoulder exercises.

1. As you press the dumbbells upward, rotate your hands so that your palms face forward.

2. Rotate back as you lower.

****

MCDONALD'S Restaurant
NIEDERHASLISTRASSE 7
8157 DIELSDORF
Tel 044 854 06 09
Hern Beat Zobrist

****

Vielen Dank für Ihren Besuch
McDonald's wünscht Ihnen einen
excellenten Appetit

****

QUITTUNG

No TVA: MWST NR 265 914#ORD 07 -REG
26/04/2010 13:27:40
ANZ PROD   TOT
  5 CA-GRILLED   49
  1 McCHIKEN   6
>>01 Nur Salat
  6 FRUIT BAG   12
  5 BALSAMICO

Take-Out Total   6
CHF
Change

TAX B (2.40%)   67.60 =

***   Oeffnungsze ten
Montag - Donnerstag :   08h30 -
Freitag und Samstag :   08h30 -
Sonntag   :   10h30 - 2

****

MCDONALD'S Restaurant
NIEDERHASLISTRASSE 7
8157 DIELSDORF
Tel 044 854 06 09
Hern Beat Zobrist

****

Vielen Dank für Ihren Besuch
McDonald's wünscht Ihnen einen
excellenten Appetit

****

QUITTUNG

No TVA: MWST NR 265 914#ORD 83 -REG 3-
24/04/2010 13:54:37
ANZ PROD
  2 CA-GRILLED   TOTAL
  1 WRAP BBQ   19.80
  2 BALSAMICO   3.90
                                   0.00
Take-Out Total
CHF   23.70
Change   24.00
                                   0.30
TAX B (2.40%)   23.70 =   0.56

***   Oeffnungszeiten
Montag - Donnerstag :   08h30 - 23h30   ***
Freitag und Samstag :   08h30 - 01h00
Sonntag   :   10h30 - 23h30

Metabolic Disturbance:

Metabolic Disturbance Training (MDT) is along the lines of cardio training, except it takes much less time (2 – 3 min warm up + 4 min actual training time) and it is much more effective for weight loss.[3]

I used 2 different protocols for my MDT : Intervals and Tabata. I did this workout most nights as it took only 6 or 7 minutes in total to do and really got my BMR (G) fired up and burning calories 24/7

Because I work in a gym I have access to all the equipment all the time. If I didn't work in a gym or was on holiday etc I would just pick one of the exercises that I could do with what I had available.

They all need some kind of timing device that lets you monitor time in seconds. For some of them that's all you need. Any digital or analog clock which indicates seconds will do, but there is an inexpensive device designed specifically for this type of training. You can read more about it on this website : www.austinfitness.ch/product.html

Intervals

This is done using any conventional aerobic activity. For the warm up I would simply perform the activity for 2 – 3 minutes starting out at a very slow pace, but increasing that pace as the warm up progressed. I would then alternate between a 20 second all out effort and a 40 second recovery period. Each cycle takes 1 minute and I would do 4 cycles.

Intervals on a Stationary Cycle - this is the easiest option and beginners should stay with this until they have developed a reasonable level of conditioning before they try any of the other options.

- Intervals on a Cross Trainer

- Intervals on a Rowing Machine

- Intervals running and walking outdoors

- Intervals can also be performed in a swimming pool

- Intervals on a Treadmill are not recommended because the machine takes too long to accelerate and decelerate and can be dangerous.

Tabata

Named after its inventor, Izumi Tabata, it is a form of interval training. With this protocol one would alternate between 20 seconds of high intensity training and 10 seconds of complete rest for a total of 4 minutes. All of the above Interval Training options could also be performed Tabata style.

Here are some additional variations I used :

📹 Dumbbell Thrusters

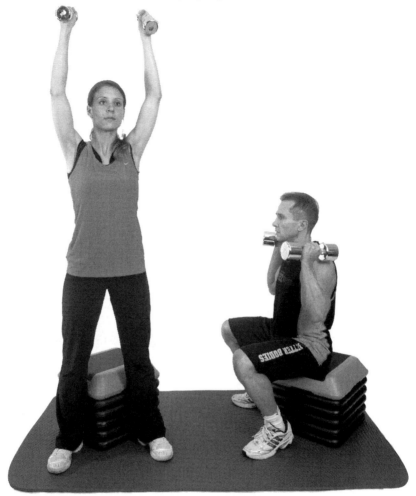

Beginners could do this with no weight and get a good workout.

I tried for 8 rounds of 12 repetitions each round, and when I could complete the 8 x 12 I would increase the weight. The new weight made me unable to do all 12 in the last 2 or 3 cycles. When I built up to the 8 x 12 again, I would increase the weight again.

📹 Jumping Squats

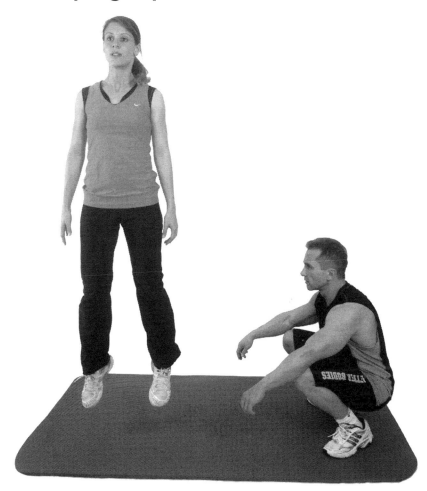

Land softly and as your feet hit the floor start to descend, decelerating as you do. In other words don't slam into the floor with straight knees, or rapidly drop down into a full squat position.

📹 Jumping Lunges

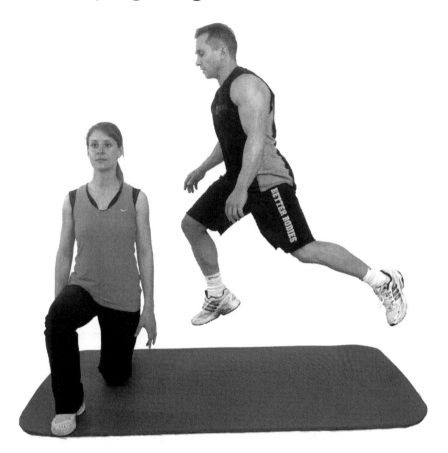

how funny is this photo . . .

Jumping Squats alternating with Jumping Lunges

Do jumping squats for 20 seconds, rest 10 seconds and then do jumping lunges for 20 seconds. Repeat this another 3 times, giving you a total of 8 intervals.

📹 Burpees

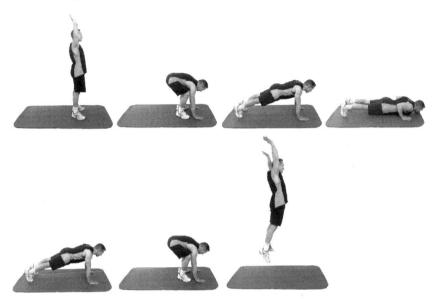

This strangely named exercise is a full body exercise with a strong cardiovascular effect . . . perfect for Tabata. And all you need for an excellent workout are a few open square feet, 4 minutes and a timer.

In case you're wondering it takes its name from an American psychologist, Royal H. Burpee who developed the Burpee test.

📷 Bulgarians

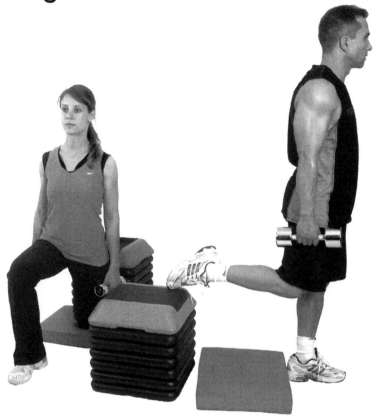

Combining Bulgarians with the Tabata Protocol is brutal and only for the most dedicated.

Do 20 seconds on one leg, rest 10 seconds and then 20 seconds on the other.

Repeat until a total of 8 rounds have been completed (4 each leg)

Jumping Rope

Surprisingly difficult, but if you are good with a skipping rope then go for it.

Steady State Cardio:

Steady State Cardio is any aerobic activity which is done at a steady pace for at least 15 to 20 minutes, but often more. The more active one is, the more calories one burns and the faster one loses weight. When time is limited, Metabolic Disturbance Training is always the favored option. But if you have the time or you enjoy steady state cardio, then in addition to MDT, one can do any of the following activities to burn extra calories.

- **Brisk walking**
- **Cycling (stationery or outdoor)**
- **Treadmill**
- **Stepper**
- **Rower**
- **Swimming**
- **Cross country skiing**

Mobility, Flexibility and Muscle Activation:

How many of these trouble you ?

• **Bad posture**

• **Occasional or regular back ache**

• **Pain in your knees, ankles, hips, shoulders, elbows or wrists**

• **Rounded shoulders**

• **Lordosis (excessive curvature of the lower back)**

• **Kyphosis (excessive curvature of the upper back, "hunch back")**

• **Poor flexibility**

The 15 minute program described at the end of this chapter improves joint mobility as well as the quality and flexibility of soft tissue (muscles, tendons and ligaments)

Running through it 3 times a week will go a long way to easing all of the above conditions and make all your daily movements far more comfortable.

Soft Tissue Release

Foam Rolling:

Years of movement, whether exercising or just every day moving around causes scar tissue and adhesions to develop in our muscles.[4] These lead to postural and movement afflictions, which in turn lead to joint damage. In other words you look, feel and move worse and worse over time. Ten minutes 3 times a week on a $20 foam roller will prevent all this and make you feel great too.

Google "foam roller" to buy one, or another option is to use

"The Stick", which is more portable, has similar results, and is easier to use for heavier people.

You can purchase the Stick by clicking on its tag on the Products tab on my website. The Original Body Stick is the most versatile option.

You will also need a baseball or some other ball similar in size and hardness.

📹 Calves

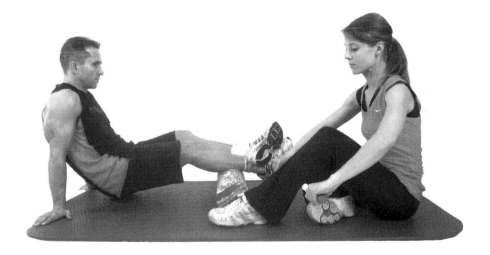

1. Stack one leg on top of the other and roll one leg at a time.

2. Keep altering your body position to reach different areas.

📹 Quadriceps

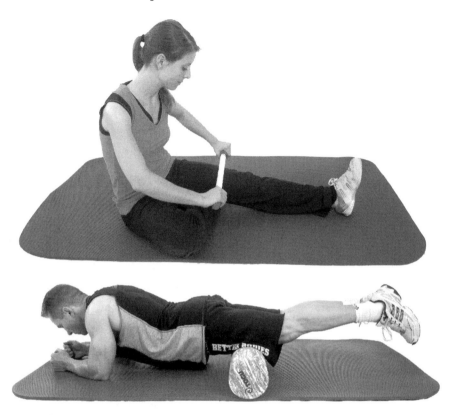

Roll back and forth from just below the hip joint to just above the knee.

📹 Progression: **Bend your knees**

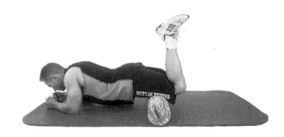

📷 Iliotibial Band

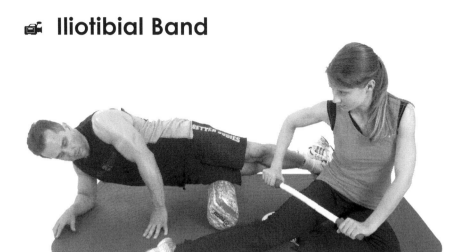

Roll back and forth from just below the hip joint to just above the knee.

📷 Buttocks

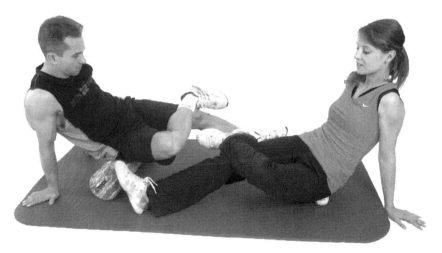

Shift your weight from one hip to the other to roll one side at a time.

◉ Hamstrings

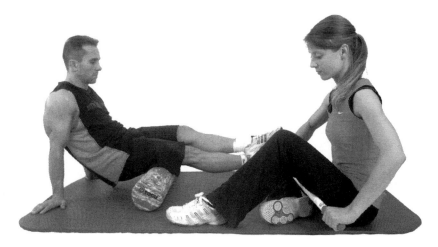

Stack one leg on top of the other and roll one leg at a time.

Roll from just under your buttocks down to just above the back of your knee.

◉ Plantar Fascia

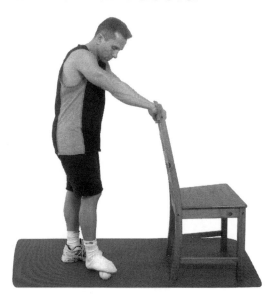

1. Put the majority of your weight on the foot that is on the ball.

2. Roll back and forth along the sole of your foot.

3. Switch feet.

Flexibility and Mobility

📹 Thoracic Spine on Foam Roller

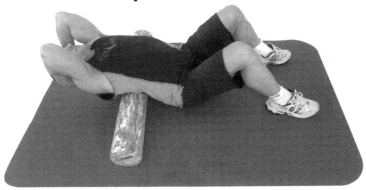

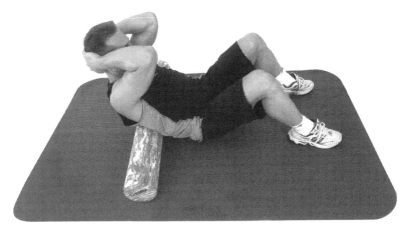

1. Your knees should be bent at 90°

2. The roller should cross your back just below your shoulder blades. Keep your elbows together, butt touching the floor and chin tucked. Do 3 repetitions and then move about 3 inches forward so the foam roller is higher up on your back and do another 3.

3. Keep moving up until the roller is about 3 inches below your neck. Do not roll your neck.

▣ Seated thoracic spine rotation

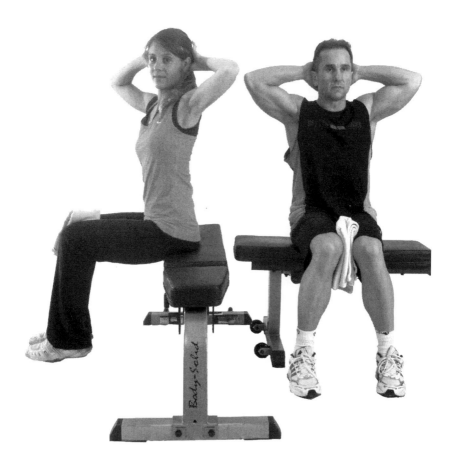

1. Grip a rolled up towel between your knees.

2. Sit up straight and tall throughout.

3. Rotate to one side keeping your abdominals braced to prevent rotation of the lower back.

4. Hold the stretch for 3 seconds.

📷 Seated 90/90

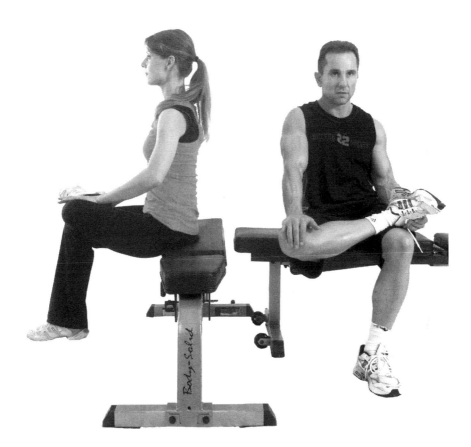

1. Keep your chest up and sit tall.

2. Press gently down just above your knee with one hand and pull up gently on your foot with the other hand.

3. Hold the stretch for about 3 seconds.

4. If you feel pain in the knee of the leg that is being stretched then reduce the range of the stretch so that you feel no pain.

📹 Lying knee to knee stretch

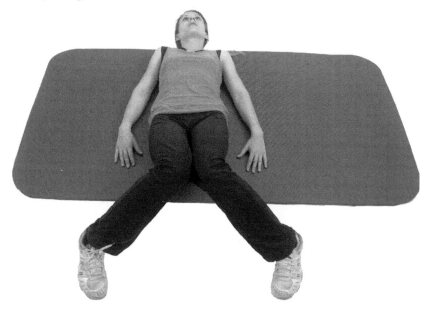

1. With feet wide apart try to touch your knees together while keeping your feet on the floor. Hold for 2 seconds and then return to the start position.

2. If you feel knee pain reduce the range of the stretch by bringing your feet closer to each other so that you feel no pain.

⌨ Supine Straight Leg Raise

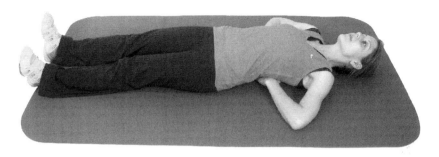

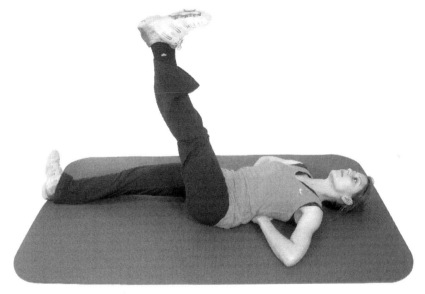

1. Keep your hands under the arch of your back.

2. Keeping both legs straight raise one leg up until you feel your back starting to push down on your hands. That's as far as you go.

3. Hold the stretch for about 3 seconds then return to start position.

4. As your hip mobility improves you should be able to get higher and higher before you feel the pressure on your hands.

📷 Kneeling Hip Flexor Stretch

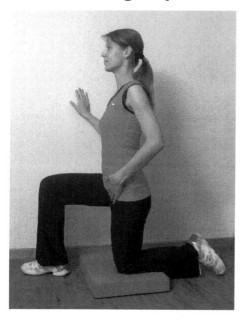

1. Make sure your feet and knees face straight ahead.

2. Keep your core tight and move forward by pushing with your buttocks muscle on the side of the knee that is down.

3. Don't arch your lower back.

📷 Progression:

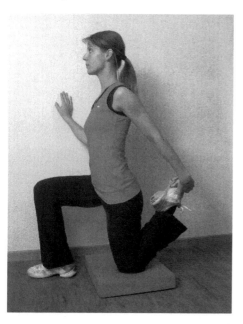

The same directions, but holding your foot with your back knee bent

☞ Ankle Mobility Drill

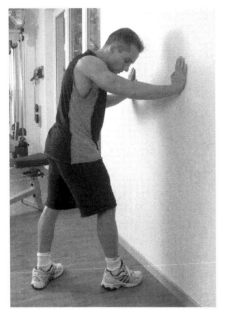 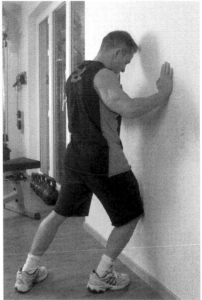

1. Start with your toes touching the wall and do 5 repetitions.

2. If you can do them comfortably with your heel firmly on the floor then increase the distance between your toes and the wall by 1 – 2 inch increments until you cannot touch the wall with your knee without lifting your heel. Remember this distance for the next time and start here.

3. Repeat 8 times each leg.

4. As your ankle mobility improves you should be able to start further from the wall.

📹 Progression:

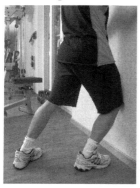 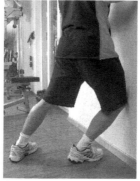 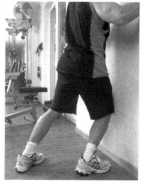

Do 5 repetitions inward, 5 directly forward and 5 outward each leg

📹 Scapular Wall Slides

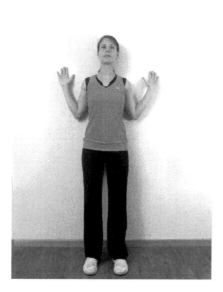 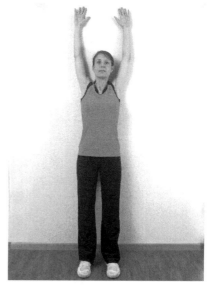

1. Stand with your heels about 6 inches away from a wall.

2. Keep your buttocks, upper back and head against the wall.

3. Slowly slide your arms up and down the wall going as far up and down as possible so you feel a stretch, but no pain.

4. Repeat 8 times.

Regression: 📹

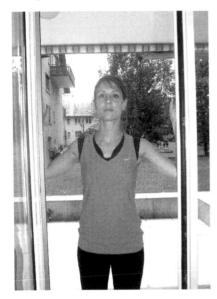

If your range is very limited or you feel pain in your shoulders with your back to the wall then stand in a doorway as far forward as you can while still getting full range. Over time you should stand further and further forward until you are able to do it with your back to the wall.

Photo shows down position

Slowly slide your arms up the door frame following the instructions for the Scapular Wall Slides above

📹 Corner Chest Stretch

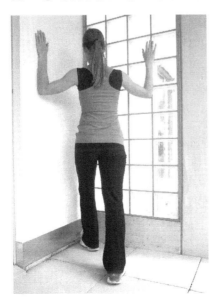

1. Elbows should be slightly below shoulder height.

2. Keep abdominals tight to avoid arching your back.

3. Lean gently in towards the corner by bending your front knee until you feel a stretch in your chest.

The Program

Foam Rolling	
Calves	Roll each calf for 30 seconds
Quadriceps	Roll for 30 seconds
Iliotibial Band	Roll each side for 30 seconds
Buttocks	Roll each side for 30 seconds
Hamstrings	Roll each leg for 30 seconds
Plantar Fascia	Roll each foot for 30 seconds

Flexibility and Mobility	
Thoracic Spine on Foam Roller	Do 3 reps in 3 different positions
Seated Thoracic Spine Rotation	Do 8 reps each side
Seated 90 / 90	Do 8 reps each side
Lying Knee to Knee Stretch	Hold the stretch for 30 seconds
Supine Straight Leg Raise	Do 8 reps each side
Kneeling Hip Flexor Stretch	Do 8 reps each side
Ankle Mobility Drill	Do 8 reps each side
Scapular Wall Slides	Do 10 reps
Corner Chest Stretch	Hold for 20 seconds then change legs

Psychology and Weight Loss

An in depth account of the role of psychology in weight loss is beyond the scope of this book. The subject includes topics like positive thinking, visualization, goal setting, self-sabotage and the like.

Without a lot of detail I will discuss two simple yet very effective techniques you can use to make sure psychology is working for, rather against you.

Over 75% of overeating is caused by emotions.[1] Overeating is usually an attempt to console oneself or to feel more comfortable or happier. The following two quick and simple exercises are proven to increase happiness without the need for food.

Gratitude Attitude

Anything you pay a lot of attention to will grow. Focusing on all the negatives or failures in your life or on what you don't have will only increase the negatives and feelings of lacking.

A 2003 study[2] showed that spending a few moments writing down things for which they were grateful or achievements they were proud of made people much happier and more optimistic. It could be getting to appreciate something in nature like a beautiful sunset or a big tree outside your window, a special friendship or relationship, or anything else in your life, circumstances or surroundings for which you are thankful. It could also be any achievement, big or small that you feel good about.

Future Perfect

Visualizing your perfect life will help bring the things you visualize into reality.

A university study[3] proved that writing about the ideal outcome for their future kept people motivated and on track, which greatly increased their rates of success. State these short sentences or affirmations in the first person present tense.

For example :

I fit into my favourite jeans comfortably

I feel light and healthy at my new weight

I look great

You will find more examples in my personal training and food intake record. And included in this book is a 30 day journal for you to record your own training and food intake, as well as space to do the above two exercises.

Should you wish to continue doing this for more than 30 days you can print further copies from my website. Go to the McDonald's Diet tab and click on "Diary"

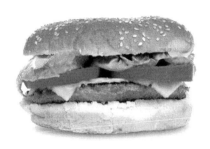

My 30 Day Diary

Mobility, Flexibility & Soft Tissue Work

Metabolic Disturbance

lower body only

Row Machine Tabata style	fast (sec)	slow (secs)	no. of intervals
Unit of Resist.	20	10	8
cal/hour	1100	300	

Strength Training

Exercise

		Weight				
1a		Reps				
1b		Weight				
		Reps				
2a		Weight				
		Reps				
2b		Weight				
		Reps				
3a		Weight				
		Reps				
3b		Weight				
		Reps				

Mind Stuff

Thankful for

having the time, health and financial freedom to conduct this experiment

Future Perfect

I am at my ideal weight.

Food and Drink Intake

	Calories
Breakfast:	
1 Fruit Bag	45
1 protein drink	150
Mid Morning	
1 Fruit Bag	45
Lunch	
1 Grilled Chicken Caesar Salad	185
1 Balsamic Dressing	25
Mid Afternoon	
1 Grilled Chicken Caesar Salad	185
1 Balsamic Dressing	25
Dinner	
1 Grilled Chicken Caesar Salad	185
1 Balsamic Dressing	25
Pre-Bed Snack	
1 Fruit Bag	45

Drinks

Sparkling Water from Mc D + filtered tap water all day long

Supplements

Omega 3 Fish Oil	45
Multivitamin and Mineral	
Total	960

Mobility, Flexibility & Soft Tissue Work

upper body only program

Metabolic Disturbance

Burpees Tabata Style	fast (sec)	slow (secs)	no. of intervals
Unit of Resist.	20	10	8
Repetitions	6	0	

Strength Training

Exercise

	Exercise					
1a	incline DB press	Weight	30	45	65	65
		Reps	12	12	10	10
1b	seated cable row	Weight	100	140	160	160
		Reps	12	12	12	12
2a	DB military press	Weight	30	45	45	45
		Reps	12	10	10	10
2b	supinated grip pulldowns	Weight	100	140	160	160
		Reps	12	12	12	12
3a		Weight				
		Reps				
3b		Weight				
		Reps				

Mind Stuff

Thankful for

loving my job

Future Perfect

I walk up stairs effortlessly

Food and Drink Intake

	Calories
Breakfast:	
1 Mc Donalds Fruit Bag	45
1 protein drink	150
Pre-Workout	
1 Mc Donalds Fruit Bag	45
Post-Workout	
1 Mc Chicken without mayo	325
Mid Afternoon	
1 Grilled Chicken Caesar Salad	185
1 Balsamic Dressing	25
Dinner	
1 Grilled Chicken Caesar Salad	185
1 Balsamic Dressing	25
Pre-Bed Snack	
1 Fruit Bag	45

Drinks

Sparkling Water from Mc D + filtered tap water all day long

Supplements

Omega 3 Fish Oil	45
Multivitamin and Mineral	
Total	1075

Mobility, Flexibility & Soft Tissue Work

upper and lower body program

Metabolic Disturbance

Burpees Tabata Style	fast (sec)	slow (secs)	no. of intervals
Unit of Resist.	20	10	8
Repetitions	5	0	

Strength Training

Exercise

1a		Weight			
		Reps			
1b		Weight			
		Reps			
2a		Weight			
		Reps			
2b		Weight			
		Reps			
3a		Weight			
		Reps			
3b		Weight			
		Reps			

Mind Stuff

Thankful for

finishing the whole set of Tabata even though I really felt like quitting half way

Future Perfect

I fit into my favorite jeans comfortably

Food and Drink Intake

	Calories
Breakfast:	
1 Fruit Bag	45
1 protein drink	150
Mid Morning	
1 Fruit Bag	45
Lunch	
1 Grilled Chicken Caesar Salad	185
1 Balsamic Dressing	25
Mid Afternoon	
1 Grilled Chicken Caesar Salad	185
1 Balsamic Dressing	25
Dinner	
6 Chicken Nuggets	250
½ BBQ Sauce	20
1 small Green Salad	10

Drinks

Sparkling Water from Mc D + filtered tap water all day long

Supplements

Omega 3 Fish Oil	45
Multivitamin and Mineral	
Total	985

Mobility, Flexibility & Soft Tissue Work

lower body only program

Metabolic Disturbance

		fast (sec)	slow (secs)	no. of intervals
jumping squat jumping lunge				
Unit of Resist.		20	10	8
Repetitions		12/20	0	

Strength Training

Exercise

	Exercise					
1a 1b 1c	Reverse Hypers 45° Back Extensions Body Weight Squats	Weight	0			
		Reps	15 each			
2a	Bird Dog with Ankle Weights	Weight	0	5	5	
		Reps	12	12	12	
2b	1 DB Goblet Squats	Weight	35	50	60	
		Reps	15	15	15	
3	2 DB Split Squats	Weight	35			
		Reps	15			
4	Prone Plank (seconds)	Weight	0			
		Reps	60			
5	Side Plank (seconds each side)	Weight	0			
		Reps	30			

Mind Stuff

Thankful for

my son having the same passion for exercise and clean living that I have

Future Perfect

all my joints feel good

Food and Drink Intake

	Calories
Breakfast:	
1 Fruit Bag	45
1 protein drink	150
Mid Morning	
1 Fruit Bag	45
Post-Workout	
1 Mc Chicken without mayo	325
Mid Afternoon	
1 Snack Wrap BBQ	275
Dinner	
1/2 Grilled Chicken Caesar Salad	93
1/2 Balsamic Dressing	12
Pre-Bed Snack	
1/2 Grilled Chicken Caesar Salad	93
1/2 Balsamic Dressing	12

Drinks

Sparkling Water from Mc D + filtered tap water all day long

Supplements

Omega 3 Fish Oil	45
Multivitamin and Mineral	
Total	1095

Mobility, Flexibility & Soft Tissue Work

leg program only

Metabolic Disturbance

Octane Crosstrainer	fast (sec)	slow (secs)	no. of intervals
Unit of Resist.	30	90	5
resist. level	85rpm level16	40rpm level13	

Strength Training

Exercise

			Weight				
1a			Reps				
1b			Weight				
			Reps				
2a			Weight				
			Reps				
2b			Weight				
			Reps				
3a			Weight				
			Reps				
3b			Weight				
			Reps				

Mind Stuff

Thankful for

living in one of the safest countries in the world

Future Perfect

I am lighter and happier

Food and Drink Intake

	Calories
Breakfast:	
1 Fruit Bag	45
1 protein drink	150
Mid Morning	
1 Fruit Bag	45
Lunch	
1 Grilled Chicken Caesar Salad	185
1 Balsamic Dressing	25
Mid Afternoon	
6 Chicken Nuggets	250
½ BBQ Sauce	20
1 small Green Salad	10
1/2 Balsamic Dressing	12
Sometime later	
1 Mc Donalds Fruit Bag 4	5
Dinner	
1 Grilled Chicken Caesar Salad	185

Drinks

Sparkling Water from Mc D + filtered tap water all day long

Supplements

Omega 3 Fish Oil	45
Multivitamin and Mineral	
Total	1017

Mobility, Flexibility & Soft Tissue Work

upper body
program only

Metabolic Disturbance

stationery cycle ergometer	fast (sec)	slow (secs)	no. of intervals
Unit of Resist.	20	40	4
Watts	500	50	

Strength Training

Exercise

1a	Decline DB Press	Weight	30	50	70	70
		Reps	12	12	10	10
1b	One Arm Cable Row	Weight	40	60	70	70
		Reps	12	12	10	10
2a	Alternating Twisting Standing DB Press	Weight	40	45	50	50
		Reps	12	12	10	10
2b	Pronated Grip Pull-downs	Weight	120	140	160	170
		Reps	12	12	12	10
3a		Weight				
		Reps				
3b		Weight				
		Reps				

Mind Stuff

Thankful for

big trees and the smell before a thunderstorm

Future Perfect

I am in total control of my eating

Food and Drink Intake

	Calories
Breakfast:	
1 protein drink	150
Mid Morning	
1 Mc Donalds Fruit Bag	45
Post-Workout	
1 Mc Chicken without mayo	325
Mid Afternoon	
1 Grilled Chicken Caesar Salad	185
Dinner	
1/2 Grilled Chicken Caesar Salad	93
1/2 Balsamic Dressing	12
Pre-Bed Snack	
1/2 Grilled Chicken Caesar Salad	93
1/2 Balsamic Dressing	12
1 Mc Donalds Fruit Bag	45

Drinks

Sparkling Water from Mc D + filtered tap water all day long

Supplements

Omega 3 Fish Oil	45
Multivitamin and Mineral	
Total	1005

Mobility, Flexibility & Soft Tissue Work

upper and lower body program

Metabolic Disturbance

	fast (sec)	slow (secs)	no. of intervals
Burpees			
Unit of Resist.	20	10	8
Repetitions	5	0	

Strength Training

Exercise

	Exercise					
1a		Weight				
		Reps				
1b		Weight				
		Reps				
2a		Weight				
		Reps				
2b		Weight				
		Reps				
3a		Weight				
		Reps				
3b		Weight				
		Reps				

Mind Stuff

Thankful for

having stuck exactly to my training and eating plan all week

Future Perfect

I wake up excited about the new day

Food and Drink Intake

	Calories
Breakfast:	
1 protein drink	150
Lunch	
1 Grilled Chicken Caesar Salad	185
1 Balsamic Dressing	25
1 Mc Donalds Fruit Bag	45
Mid Afternoon	
1 Grilled Chicken Caesar Salad	185
1 Balsamic Dressing	25
Sometime Later	
1 Mc Donalds Fruit Bag	45
Dinner	
1 Grilled Chicken Caesar Salad	185
1 Balsamic Dressing	25

Drinks

Sparkling Water from Mc D + filtered tap water all day long

Supplements

Omega 3 Fish Oil	45
Multivitamin and Mineral	
Total	915

Mobility, Flexibility & Soft Tissue Work

lower body program

Metabolic Disturbance

	fast (sec)	slow (secs)	no. of intervals
Unit of Resist.			

Strength Training

Exercise

	Exercise					
1a 1b 1c	Reverse Hypers 45° Back Extensions Body Weight Squats	Weight	0			
		Reps	15 each			
2a	Romanian Deadlift	Weight	90	155	200	
		Reps	12	12	12	
2b	1 DB Goblet Squats	Weight	30	55	65	
		Reps	12	12	12	
2c	DB Reverse Lunge from Deficit (reps per leg)	Weight	30	35		
		Reps	8	8		
3a	Mc Gill Crunch	Weight	0	0		
		Reps	2x12	2x12		
3b	Incline Prone Plank (seconds)	Weight	0	0		
		Reps	60	60		

Mind Stuff

Thankful for

my first 5 pounds of fat already gone

Future Perfect

I am strong and have a kick-ass body

Food and Drink Intake

	Calories
Breakfast:	
1 protein drink	150
1 Mc Donalds Fruit Bag	45
Mid Morning	
1 Grilled Chicken Caesar Salad	185
1 Balsamic Dressing	25
Pre Workout	
1 Mc Donalds Fruit Bag	45
1 Mc Chicken without mayo	325
Mid Afternoon	
1 Grilled Chicken Caesar Salad	185
1 Balsamic Dressing	25
Dinner	
1 Grilled Chicken Caesar Salad	185
1 Balsamic Dressing	25

Drinks

Sparkling Water from Mc D + filtered tap water all day long

Supplements

Omega 3 Fish Oil	45
Multivitamin and Mineral	
Total	1240

Mobility, Flexibility & Soft Tissue Work

lower body program

Metabolic Disturbance

jumping squat jumping lunge	fast (sec)	slow (secs)	no. of intervals
Unit of Resist.	20	10	8
repetitions	12/20	0	

Strength Training

Exercise

1a	Weight				
	Reps				
1b	Weight				
	Reps				
2a	Weight				
	Reps				
2b	Weight				
	Reps				
3a	Weight				
	Reps				
3b	Weight				
	Reps				

Mind Stuff

Thankful for

getting a massage

Future Perfect

I buy clothes that emphasise my appearance

Food and Drink Intake

	Calories
Breakfast:	
1 protein drink	150
1 Mc Donalds Fruit Bag	45
Lunch	
1 Grilled Chicken Caesar Salad	185
1 Balsamic Dressing	25
Mid Afternoon	
1 Grilled Chicken Caesar Salad	185
1 Balsamic Dressing	25
Sometime Later	
1 Mc Donalds Fruit Bag	45
Dinner	
1 Grilled Chicken Caesar Salad	185
1 Balsamic Dressing	25

Drinks

Sparkling Water from Mc D + filtered tap water all day long

Supplements

Omega 3 Fish Oil	45
Multivitamin and Mineral	
Total	915

Mobility, Flexibility & Soft Tissue Work

only upper body

Metabolic Disturbance

rope jumping	fast (sec)	slow (secs)	no. of intervals
Unit of Resist.	20	10	8
not applicable			

Strength Training

Exercise

	Exercise					
1a	weighted incline push-ups on stands	Weight	0	45	45	45
		Reps	12	12	10	10
1b	2 point bent over one arm DB Row	Weight	35	50	65	65
		Reps	12	12	12	12
2a	Seated Arnold Press	Weight	30	45	45	45
		Reps	12	12	10	7
2b	Pronated Grip Pull-ups	Weight	0	0	0	0
		Reps	12	12	10	9
3a		Weight				
		Reps				
3b		Weight				
		Reps				

Mind Stuff

Thankful for

the walk home from work every evening which gives me fresh air, solitude and a chance to reflect on my day

Future Perfect

I enjoy exercising regularly

Food and Drink Intake

	Calories
Breakfast:	
1 protein drink	150
Pre-Workout	
1 Mc Donalds Fruit Bag	45
Post-Workout	
1 Mc Chicken without mayo	325
Mid Afternoon	
1 Grilled Chicken Caesar Salad	185
1 Balsamic Dressing	25
Dinner	
1 Grilled Chicken Caesar Salad	185
1 Balsamic Dressing	25

Drinks

Sparkling Water from Mc D + filtered tap water all day long

Supplements

Omega 3 Fish Oil	45
Multivitamin and Mineral	
Total	985

Mobility, Flexibility & Soft Tissue Work

upper and lower body program

Metabolic Disturbance

jumping squat jumping lunge	fast (sec)	slow (secs)	no. of intervals
Unit of Resist.	20	10	8
repetitions	12/20	0	

Strength Training

Exercise

		Weight				
1a		Reps				
1b		Weight				
		Reps				
2a		Weight				
		Reps				
2b		Weight				
		Reps				
3a		Weight				
		Reps				
3b		Weight				
		Reps				

Mind Stuff

Thankful for

I make a comfortable living doing what I love

Future Perfect

I go to sleep each night proud of my progress for the day

Food and Drink Intake

	Calories
Breakfast:	
1 protein drink	150
1 Mc Donalds Fruit Bag	45
Mid Morning	
1 Mc Donalds Fruit Bag	45
Lunch	
McWrap Grilled Chicken	410
Mid Afternoon	
1 Grilled Chicken Caesar Salad	185
1 Balsamic Dressing	25
Sometime later	
1 Mc Donalds Fruit Bag	45
Dinner	
1 Grilled Chicken Caesar Salad	185
1 Balsamic Dressing	25
Pre-Bed Snack	
1/3 McWrap Grilled Chicken	136

Drinks

Sparkling Water from Mc D + filtered tap water all day long

Supplements

Omega 3 Fish Oil	45
Multivitamin and Mineral	
Total	1296

Mobility, Flexibility & Soft Tissue Work

upper and lower body program

Metabolic Disturbance

Octane Crosstrainer	fast (sec)	slow (secs)	no. of intervals
Unit of Resist.	30	90	5
resist. level	85rpm level16	40rpm level13	

Strength Training

Exercise

	Exercise		Weight				
1a		Weight					
		Reps					
1b		Weight					
		Reps					
2a		Weight					
		Reps					
2b		Weight					
		Reps					
3a		Weight					
		Reps					
3b		Weight					
		Reps					

Mind Stuff

Thankful for

my parents' infinite support

Future Perfect

I only eat what I need

Food and Drink Intake

	Calories
Breakfast:	
1 protein drink	150
1 Mc Donalds Fruit Bag	45
Mid Morning	
1 Mc Donalds Fruit Bag	45
Lunch	
1 Grilled Chicken Caesar Salad	185
1 Balsamic Dressing	25
A Little Later	
1 Mc Donalds Fruit Bag	45
Mid Afternoon	
1 Grilled Chicken Caesar Salad	185
A Little Later	
1 Mc Donalds Fruit Bag	45
Dinner	
1 Grilled Chicken Caesar Salad	185
1 Balsamic Dressing	25

Drinks

Sparkling Water from Mc D + filtered tap water all day long

Supplements

Omega 3 Fish Oil	45
Multivitamin and Mineral	
Total	980

Mobility, Flexibility & Soft Tissue Work

lower body only

Metabolic Disturbance

	fast (sec)	slow (secs)	no. of intervals
Unit of Resist.			

Strength Training

Exercise

1a 1b 1c	Bodyweight Squats Reverse Hypers 45° Back Extensions	Weight Reps	30 15 15		
2a	Sumo Style Romanian Deadlift	Weight	90	155	180
		Reps	12	12	12
2b	BB Front Squat	Weight	70	130	150
		Reps	6	6	6
2c	DB Bulgarian Split Squats	Weight	35	50	65
		Reps	8	8	8
3a	Mc Gill Crunch	Weight	2 x 12		
3b	Weighted Side Plank	Reps	60		
3b	Side Plank with DB Resting on Top Leg	Weight	10		
		Reps	30		

Mind Stuff

Thankful for — big bear hugs from my brother

Future Perfect — I am a great example to my kids and my family

Food and Drink Intake

Food and Drink Intake	Calories
Breakfast:	
1 protein drink	150
Pre-Workout	
1 Mc Donalds Fruit Bag	45
Post-Workout	
1 Mc Chicken without mayo	325
Mid Afternoon	
1 Grilled Chicken Caesar Salad without dressing	185
1 Mc Donalds Fruit Bag	45
Sometime later	
1 Mc Donalds Fruit Bag	45
Dinner	
1 Grilled Chicken Caesar Salad	185
1 Balsamic Dressing	25

Drinks

Sparkling Water from Mc D + filtered tap water all day long

Supplements

Omega 3 Fish Oil	45
Multivitamin and Mineral	
Total	1050

Mobility, Flexibility & Soft Tissue Work

Metabolic Disturbance

	upper and lower program

jumping squat jumping lunge	fast (sec)	slow (secs)	no. of intervals
Unit of Resist.	20	10	8
repetitions	12/20	0	

Strength Training

Exercise

	Exercise		Set 1	Set 2	Set 3	Set 4
1a		Weight				
		Reps				
1b		Weight				
		Reps				
2a		Weight				
		Reps				
2b		Weight				
		Reps				
3a		Weight				
		Reps				
3b		Weight				
		Reps				

Mind Stuff

Thankful for — driving on a warm night with the top down

Future Perfect — I jog for fun

Food and Drink Intake

	Calories
Breakfast:	
1 protein drink	150
1 Mc Donalds Fruit Bag	45
Mid Morning	
1 Mc Donalds Fruit Bag	45
Lunch	
1 Grilled Chicken Caesar Salad	185
1 Balsamic Dressing	25
A Little Later	
1 Mc Donalds Fruit Bag	45
Mid Afternoon	
1 Grilled Chicken Caesar Salad	185
1 Balsamic Dressing	25
Sometime later	
1 Mc Donalds Fruit Bag	45
Dinner	
1 Grilled Chicken Caesar Salad	185
1 Balsamic Dressing	25
A Little Later	
1 Mc Donalds Fruit Bag	45

Drinks

Sparkling Water from Mc D + filtered tap water all day long

Supplements

Omega 3 Fish Oil	45
Multivitamin and Mineral	
Total	1050

Mobility, Flexibility & Soft Tissue Work

Metabolic Disturbance

	fast (sec)	slow (secs)	no. of intervals
Unit of Resist.			

Strength Training

Exercise

	Exercise		Set 1	Set 2	Set 3	Set 4
1a		Weight				
		Reps				
1b		Weight				
		Reps				
2a		Weight				
		Reps				
2b		Weight				
		Reps				
3a		Weight				
		Reps				
3b		Weight				
		Reps				

Mind Stuff

Thankful for

watching a snow storm outside

Future Perfect

all my clothes are loose on me

Food and Drink Intake

	Calories
Breakfast:	
1 protein drink	150
1 Mc Donalds Fruit Bag	45
Mid Morning	
1 Mc Donalds Fruit Bag	45
Lunch	
1 Grilled Chicken Caesar Salad	185
1 Balsamic Dressing	25
Mid Afternoon	
1 Grilled Chicken Caesar Salad	185
1 Balsamic Dressing	25
Dinner	
1 Grilled Chicken Caesar Salad	185
1 Balsamic Dressing	25
Before Bed	
1 Mc Donalds Fruit Bag	45

Drinks

Sparkling Water from Mc D + filtered tap water all day long

Supplements

Omega 3 Fish Oil	45
Multivitamin and Mineral	
Total	960

Mobility, Flexibility & Soft Tissue Work

upper body program

Metabolic Disturbance

Dumbbell Thrusters	fast (sec)	slow (secs)	no. of intervals
Unit of Resist.	20	10	8
pounds/ DB	15	0	

Strength Training

Exercise

	Exercise					
1a	Neutral Grip DB Military Press	Weight	30	45	45	50
		Reps	12	12	12	12
1b	Supinated Grip Pull-ups	Weight	0	45	45	45
		Reps	12	8	8	8
1c	Weighted Incline Push-ups on Stands	Weight	45	45	45	45
		Reps	12	12	12	9
1d	Weighted Horizontal Pull-ups with feet raised	Weight	45	45	45	45
		Reps	12	10	9	9
		Weight				
		Reps				
		Weight				
		Reps				

Mind Stuff

Thankful for

the Internet and text messaging

Future Perfect

my six pack abs are showing

Food and Drink Intake

	Calories
Breakfast:	
1 protein drink	150
1 Mc Donalds Fruit Bag	45
Pre-Workout	
1 Mc Donalds Fruit Bag	45
Post-Workout	
1 1/2 Fillit o Fish burgers without sauce	490
Mid Afternoon	
1 Grilled Chicken Caesar Salad	185
1 Balsamic Dressing	25
1 Mc Donalds Fruit Bag	45
Dinner	
1 Grilled Chicken Caesar Salad	185
1 Balsamic Dressing	25
Before Bed	
1 Mc Donalds Fruit Bag	45

Drinks

Sparkling Water from Mc D + filtered tap water all day long

Supplements

Omega 3 Fish Oil	45
Multivitamin and Mineral	
Total	1285

Mobility, Flexibility & Soft Tissue Work

lower body only

Metabolic Disturbance

Dumbbell Thrusters	fast (sec)	slow (secs)	no. of intervals
Unit of Resist.	20	10	8
pounds/ DB	17	0	

Strength Training

Exercise

	Exercise		Weight				
1a		Weight					
		Reps					
1b		Weight					
		Reps					
2a		Weight					
		Reps					
2b		Weight					
		Reps					
3a		Weight					
		Reps					
3b		Weight					
		Reps					

Mind Stuff

Thankful for

having a job helping people all day long

Future Perfect

my appearance is one of my strong points

Food and Drink Intake

	Calories
Breakfast:	
1 protein drink	150
1 Mc Donalds Fruit Bag	45
Lunch	
1 Grilled Chicken Caesar Salad	185
1 Balsamic Dressing	25
Mid Afternoon	
1 Grilled Chicken Caesar Salad	185
1 Balsamic Dressing	25
1 Fruit Bag	45
Dinner	
1 Grilled Chicken Caesar Salad	185
1 Balsamic Dressing	25
Before Bed	
1 Mc Donalds Fruit Bag	45

Drinks

Sparkling Water from Mc D + filtered tap water all day long

Supplements

Omega 3 Fish Oil	45
Multivitamin and Mineral	
Total	960

Mobility, Flexibility & Soft Tissue Work

lower body only

Metabolic Disturbance

	fast (sec)	slow (secs)	no. of intervals
Unit of Resist.			

Strength Training

Exercise

	Exercise					
1a 1b 1c	Bodyweight Squats Reverse Hypers 45 ° Back Extensions	Weight Reps	30 15 15			
2a	Sumo Style Romanian Deadlift	Weight	90	155	185	
		Reps	12	12	12	
2b	BB Front Squat	Weight	70	130	150	
		Reps	6	6	6	
2c	2 DB Reverse Lunge to a deficit	Weight	40	45		
		Reps	8	8		
3	Ab Wheel Rollouts	Weight	0	0	0	
		Reps	10	10	10	
4	Palloff Press	Weight	20	25	25	
		Reps	3 x 10 seconds per set			

Mind Stuff

Thankful for

every one of the more than 1,000 workouts I had with Reg Park

Future Perfect

any day that I can train is a good day

Food and Drink Intake

	Calories
Breakfast:	
1 protein drink	150
1 Mc Donalds Fruit Bag	45
Pre-Workout	
1 Mc Donalds Fruit Bag	45
Post-Workout	
1 1/2 Fillit o Fish burger without sauce	490
Lunch	
1 Grilled Chicken Caesar Salad	185
1 Balsamic Dressing	25
1 Mc Donalds Fruit Bag	45
Mid Afternoon	
1 Grilled Chicken Caesar Salad	185
1 Balsamic Dressing	25
1 Mc Donalds Fruit Bag	45
Dinner	
1 Grilled Chicken Caesar Salad	185
1 Balsamic Dressing	25
Before Bed	
1 Mc Donalds Fruit Bag	45

Drinks

Sparkling Water from Mc D + filtered tap water all day long

Supplements

Omega 3 Fish Oil	45
Multivitamin and Mineral	
Total	1540

Mobility, Flexibility & Soft Tissue Work

lower body only

Metabolic Disturbance

	fast (sec)	slow (secs)	no. of intervals
jumping squat jumping lunge			
Unit of Resist.	20	10	8
repetitions	12/20	0	

Strength Training

Exercise

1a		Weight			
		Reps			
1b		Weight			
		Reps			
2a		Weight			
		Reps			
2b		Weight			
		Reps			
3a		Weight			
		Reps			
3b		Weight			
		Reps			

Mind Stuff

Thankful for

Mozart, Bruce Springsteen and great movies

Future Perfect

it is easy for me to follow a healthy eating plan

Food and Drink Intake

	Calories
Breakfast:	
1 protein drink	150
1 Mc Donalds Fruit Bag	45
Lunch	
1 Grilled Chicken Caesar Salad	185
1 Balsamic Dressing	25
Mid Afternoon	
1 Grilled Chicken Caesar Salad	185
1 Balsamic Dressing	25
Sometime later	
1 Mc Donalds Fruit Bag	45
Dinner	
1 Grilled Chicken Caesar Salad	185
1 Balsamic Dressing	25
A Little Later	
1 Mc Donalds Fruit Bag	45

Drinks

Sparkling Water from Mc D + filtered tap water all day long

Supplements

Omega 3 Fish Oil	45
Multivitamin and Mineral	
Total	960

Mobility, Flexibility & Soft Tissue Work

Metabolic Disturbance

lower body only

jumping squat jumping lunge	fast (sec)	slow (secs)	no. of intervals
Unit of Resist.	20	10	8
repetitions	12/20	0	

Strength Training

Exercise

	Exercise					
1a	Neutral Grip DB Military Press	Weight	30	50	55	55
		Reps	8	8	8	9
1b	Supinated Grip Pull-ups	Weight	0	50	50	50
		Reps	8	8	8	6
1c	Weighted Incline Push-ups on Stands	Weight	0	50	50	50
		Reps	8	8	8	9
1d	Weighted Horizontal Pull-ups with feet raised	Weight	0	50	50	50
		Reps	8	8	8	8
		Weight				
		Reps				
		Weight				
		Reps				

Mind Stuff

Thankful for

living in a small town surrounded by the beauty of nature

Future Perfect

I love the way I look

Food and Drink Intake

	Calories
Breakfast:	
1 protein drink	150
Pre-Workout	
1 Mc Donalds Fruit Bag	45
Post-Workout	
McWrap Grilled Chicken	410
Mid Afternoon	
1 Grilled Chicken Caesar Salad without dressing	185
1 Mc Donalds Fruit Bag	45
Sometime later	
1 Mc Donalds Fruit Bag	45
Dinner	
1 Grilled Chicken Caesar Salad	185
1 Balsamic Dressing	25
Before Bed	
1 Mc Donalds Fruit Bag	45

Drinks

Sparkling Water from Mc D + filtered tap water all day long

Supplements

Omega 3 Fish Oil	45
Multivitamin and Mineral	
Total	1180

The McDonald's Diet Daily Training Record

Mobility, Flexibility & Soft Tissue Work

Metabolic Disturbance

	fast (sec)	slow (secs)	no. of intervals
Unit of Resist.			

Strength Training

Exercise

		Weight				
1a		Weight				
		Reps				
1b		Weight				
		Reps				
2a		Weight				
		Reps				
2b		Weight				
		Reps				
3a		Weight				
		Reps				
3b		Weight				
		Reps				

Mind Stuff

Thankful for

dishwashing machines

Future Perfect

I enjoy eating the foods that make me thin

Food and Drink Intake

	Calories
Breakfast:	
1 protein drink	150
1 Fruit Bag	45
Mid Morning	
1 Fruit Bag	45
Lunch	
1 Grilled Chicken Caesar Salad	185
1 Balsamic Dressing	25
Mid Afternoon	
1 Grilled Chicken Caesar Salad	185
1 Balsamic Dressing	25
At the Movies	
2 Mc Donalds Fruit Bag	90
1 sparkling McWater	0
Dinner	
1 Grilled Chicken Caesar Salad	185
1 Balsamic Dressing	25
A Little Later	
1 Mc Donalds Fruit Bag	45

Drinks

Sparkling Water from Mc D + filtered tap water all day long

Supplements

Omega 3 Fish Oil	45
Multivitamin and Mineral	
Total	1050

The McDonald's Diet Daily Training Record

Mobility, Flexibility & Soft Tissue Work

upper body

Metabolic Disturbance

intervals on rowing m/c	fast (sec)	slow (secs)	no. of intervals
Unit of Resist.	30	90	6
watts	1300	500	

Strength Training

Exercise

	Exercise					
1a		Weight				
		Reps				
1b		Weight				
		Reps				
2a		Weight				
		Reps				
2b		Weight				
		Reps				
3a		Weight				
		Reps				
3b		Weight				
		Reps				

Mind Stuff

Thankful for

salad

Future Perfect

when I look in the mirror
I am happy with what I see

Food and Drink Intake

	Calories
Breakfast:	
1 protein drink	150
1 Fruit Bag	45
Mid Morning	
1 Fruit Bag	45
Lunch	
1 Grilled Chicken Caesar Salad	185
1 Balsamic Dressing	25
Mid Afternoon	
1 Grilled Chicken Caesar Salad	185
1 Balsamic Dressing	25
Dinner	
1 Grilled Chicken Caesar Salad	185
1 Balsamic Dressing	25
1 Fruit Bag	45

Drinks

Sparkling Water from Mc D + filtered tap water all day long

Supplements

Omega 3 Fish Oil	45
Multivitamin and Mineral	
Total	960

Mobility, Flexibility & Soft Tissue Work

lower body

Metabolic Disturbance

	fast (sec)	slow (secs)	no. of intervals
Unit of Resist.			

Strength Training

Exercise

	Exercise		fast	slow	no.	
1a 1b 1c	Bodyweight Squats Reverse Hypers 45 ° Back Extensions	Weight Reps	20 10 10			
2a	BB Romanian Deadlift	Weight	90	155	220	
		Reps	10	10	10	
2b	BB Bulgarian Split Squats	Weight	65	90	120	
		Reps	10	10	10	
2c	Kettlebell Goblet Squats	Weight	45	70	70	
		Reps	10	10	10	
3	Ab Wheel Rollouts	Weight	0	0	0	
		Reps	10	10	10	
4	Palloff Press	Weight	20	25	25	
		Reps	3 x 10 seconds per set			

Mind Stuff

Thankful for

sunsets

Future Perfect

I am full of energy and vitality

Food and Drink Intake

	Calories
Breakfast:	
1 protein drink	150
1 Fruit Bag	45
Pre-Workout	
1 Mc Donalds Fruit Bag	45
Post-Workout	
1 Mc Chicken without mayo	325
shared half a shrimps	165
Mid Afternoon	
1 Grilled Chicken Caesar Salad	185
1 Balsamic Dressing	25
Dinner	
1 Grilled Chicken Caesar Salad	185
1 Balsamic Dressing	25
Before Bed	
1 Mc Donalds Fruit Bag	45

Drinks

Sparkling Water from Mc D + filtered tap water all day long

Supplements

Omega 3 Fish Oil	45
Multivitamin and Mineral	
Total	1240

The McDonald's Diet Daily Training Record

Mobility, Flexibility & Soft Tissue Work

lower body

Metabolic Disturbance

	fast (sec)	slow (secs)	no. of intervals
jumping squat jumping lunge			
Unit of Resist.	20	10	8
repetitions	15/20	0	

Strength Training

Exercise

1a	Weight				
	Reps				
1b	Weight				
	Reps				
2a	Weight				
	Reps				
2b	Weight				
	Reps				
3a	Weight				
	Reps				
3b	Weight				
	Reps				

Mind Stuff

Thankful for

my family

Future Perfect

I fit comfortably into all my slim clothes

Food and Drink Intake

	Calories
Breakfast:	
1 protein drink	150
1 Fruit Bag	45
Mid Morning	
1 Fruit Bag	45
Lunch	
1 Grilled Chicken Caesar Salad	185
1 Balsamic Dressing	25
Mid Afternoon	
1 Grilled Chicken Caesar Salad	185
1 Balsamic Dressing	25
Sometime Later	
1 Fruit Bag	45
Dinner	
1 Grilled Chicken Caesar Salad	185
1 Balsamic Dressing	25
1 Fruit Bag	45

Drinks

Sparkling Water from Mc D + filtered tap water all day long

Supplements

Omega 3 Fish Oil	45
Multivitamin and Mineral	
Total	1005

Mobility, Flexibility & Soft Tissue Work

Metabolic Disturbance

	upper body program

intervals on rowing m/c	fast (sec)	slow (secs)	no. of intervals
Unit of Resist.	30	90	6
watts	1300	500	

Strength Training

Exercise

	Exercise					
1a	Flat Barbell Press	Weight	65	110	155	165
		Reps	8	8	8	8
1b	Weighted Neutral Grip Pull-ups	Weight	0	20	45	65
		Reps	8	8	8	7
2a	Alternating Pronating Standing DB Press	Weight	35	55	55	55
		Reps	8	8	8	8
2b	Three Point One Arm DB Row	Weight	45	70	90	90
		Reps	8	8	8	8
3a		Weight				
		Reps				
3b		Weight				
		Reps				

Mind Stuff

Thankful for

being able to stay in a nice hotel when I take a holiday

Future Perfect

I maintain my ideal weight easily

Food and Drink Intake

	Calories
Breakfast:	
1 protein drink	150
1 Fruit Bag	45
Pre-Workout	
1 Mc Donalds Fruit Bag	45
Post-Workout	
1 Mc Chicken without mayo	325
Mid Afternoon	
1 Grilled Chicken Caesar Salad	185
1 Balsamic Dressing	25
Sometime Later	
1 Fruit Bag	45
Dinner	
1 Grilled Chicken Caesar Salad	185
Balsamic Dressing	25

Drinks

Sparkling Water from Mc D + filtered tap water all day long

Supplements

Omega 3 Fish Oil	45
Multivitamin and Mineral	
Total	1075

Mobility, Flexibility & Soft Tissue Work

lower body

Metabolic Disturbance

Burpees	fast (sec)	slow (secs)	no. of intervals
Unit of Resist.	20	10	8
Repetitions	7	0	

Strength Training

Exercise

	Exercise		Weight				
1a			Weight				
			Reps				
1b			Weight				
			Reps				
2a			Weight				
			Reps				
2b			Weight				
			Reps				
3a			Weight				
			Reps				
3b			Weight				
			Reps				

Mind Stuff

Thankful for

> the high that goes with accomplishment

Future Perfect

> I enjoy participating in sport

Food and Drink Intake

	Calories
Breakfast:	
1 protein drink	150
1 Fruit Bag	45
Lunch	
McWrap Grilled Chicken	410
Mid Afternoon	
1 Grilled Chicken Caesar Salad	185
1 Balsamic Dressing	25
Sometime Later	
1 Fruit Bag	45
Dinner	
1 Grilled Chicken Caesar Salad	185
1 Balsamic Dressing	25

Drinks

Sparkling Water from Mc D + filtered tap water all day long

Supplements

Omega 3 Fish Oil	45
Multivitamin and Mineral	
Total	1115

Mobility, Flexibility & Soft Tissue Work

lower body	

Metabolic Disturbance

	jumping squat jumping lunge	fast (sec)	slow (secs)	no. of intervals
Unit of Resist.		20	10	8
Repetitions		15/20	0	

Strength Training

Exercise

	Exercise					
1a	Body Weight Squats	Weight	30			
1b	45° Back Extensions	Reps	12			
2a	Sumo Grip Romanian Deadlift	Weight	90	155	220	240
		Reps	8	8	8	8
2b	KB Goblet Squat (at the moment I don't have a heavier Kettlebell)	Weight	60	70	70	
		Reps	12	12	12	12
2c	BB Bulgarian Split Squats	Weight	65	110	130	
		Reps	8	8	8	
3a	Ab Wheel Rollouts	Weight	0	0		
		Reps	10	10		
3b	McGill Crunches	Weight	0	0		
		Reps	12	12		

Mind Stuff

Thankful for

Sunday lunches at mom with the whole family

Future Perfect

I can do strenuous physical stuff with the kids without getting out of breath or injured

Food and Drink Intake

	Calories
Breakfast:	
1 protein drink	150
1 Fruit Bag	45
Pre-Workout	
1 Mc Donalds Fruit Bag	45
Post-Workout	
1 Mc Chicken without mayo	325
Mid Afternoon	
1 Grilled Chicken Caesar Salad	185
1 Balsamic Dressing	25
Dinner	
1 Grilled Chicken Caesar Salad	185
1 Balsamic Dressing	25

Drinks

Sparkling Water from Mc D + filtered tap water all day long

Supplements

Omega 3 Fish Oil	45
Multivitamin and Mineral	
Total	1030

Mobility, Flexibility & Soft Tissue Work

lower body

Metabolic Disturbance

Octane Crosstrainer	fast (sec)	slow (secs)	no. of intervals
Unit of Resist.	20	40	5
% Max HR	92	85	

Strength Training

Exercise

		Weight				
1a		Weight				
		Reps				
1b		Weight				
		Reps				
2a		Weight				
		Reps				
2b		Weight				
		Reps				
3a		Weight				
		Reps				
3b		Weight				
		Reps				

Mind Stuff

Thankful for

the starry sky on a clear night in the countryside

Future Perfect

training is my favorite activity of the day

Food and Drink Intake

	Calories
Breakfast:	
1 protein drink	150
1 Fruit Bag	45
Lunch	
1 Grilled Chicken Caesar Salad	185
1 Balsamic Dressing	25
Mid Afternoon	
1 Grilled Chicken Caesar Salad	185
1 Balsamic Dressing	25
Sometime Later	
1 Fruit Bag	45
Dinner	
1 Grilled Chicken Caesar Salad	185
1 Balsamic Dressing	25

Drinks

Sparkling Water from Mc D + filtered tap water all day long

Supplements

Omega 3 Fish Oil	45
Multivitamin and Mineral	
Total	915

Mobility, Flexibility & Soft Tissue Work

Metabolic Disturbance

	fast (sec)	slow (secs)	no. of intervals
Unit of Resist.			

Strength Training

Exercise

1a		Weight				
		Reps				
1b		Weight				
		Reps				
2a		Weight				
		Reps				
2b		Weight				
		Reps				
3a		Weight				
		Reps				
3b		Weight				
		Reps				

Mind Stuff

Thankful for

compliments from a stranger

Future Perfect

jealous overweight people tell me I am too thin now and I shouldn't lose any more weight

Food and Drink Intake

	Calories
Breakfast:	
1 protein drink	150
1 Fruit Bag	45
Lunch	
1 Grilled Chicken Caesar Salad	185
1 Balsamic Dressing	25
Mid Afternoon	
9 Chicken nuggets (slightly off plan :-( )	380
1 curry sauce	40
Dinner	
1 Grilled Chicken Caesar Salad	185
1 Balsamic Dressing	25
1 Fruit Bag	45

Drinks

Sparkling Water from Mc D + filtered tap water all day long

Supplements

Omega 3 Fish Oil	45
Multivitamin and Mineral	
Total	1125

Mobility, Flexibility & Soft Tissue Work

Metabolic Disturbance

Burpees	fast (sec)	slow (secs)	no. of intervals
Unit of Resist.	20	10	8
Repetitions	7	0	

upper body

Strength Training

Exercise

	Exercise					
1a	incline DB Press	Weight	40	55	70	70
		Reps	8	8	8	8
1b	Neutral Grip Weighted Pull-ups	Weight	0	45	65	65
		Reps	8	8	8	7
2a	Alternating Pronating Standing DB Press	Weight	35	45	55	65
		Reps	8	8	8	7
2b	1 Arm Cable Row	Weight	40	60	80	80
		Reps	8	8	8	8
3a		Weight				
		Reps				
3b		Weight				
		Reps				

Mind Stuff

Thankful for

a future wide open

Future Perfect

my body is stronger, slimmer and healthier than ever before

Food and Drink Intake

	Calories
Breakfast:	
1 protein drink	150
1 Fruit Bag	45
Pre-Workout	
1 Mc Donalds Fruit Bag	45
Post-Workout	
1 Mc Chicken without mayo	325
Mid Afternoon	
1 Grilled Chicken Caesar Salad	185
1 Balsamic Dressing	25
Dinner	
1 Grilled Chicken Caesar Salad	185
1 Balsamic Dressing	25

Drinks

Sparkling Water from Mc D + filtered tap water all day long

Supplements

Omega 3 Fish Oil	45
Multivitamin and Mineral	
Total	1030

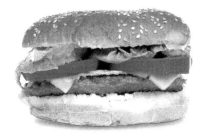

Your 30 Day Diary

Mobility, Flexibility & Soft Tissue Work

Metabolic Disturbance

	fast (sec)	slow (secs)	no. of intervals
Unit of Resist.			

Strength Training

Exercise

	Weight			
	Reps			
	Weight			
	Reps			
	Weight			
	Reps			
	Weight			
	Reps			
	Weight			
	Reps			
	Weight			
	Reps			

Mind Stuff

Thankful for

Future Perfect

Food and Drink Intake

Calories

Drinks

Supplements

Total	

Mobility, Flexibility & Soft Tissue Work

Metabolic Disturbance

	fast (sec)	slow (secs)	no. of intervals
Unit of Resist.			

Strength Training

Exercise

Exercise					
	Weight				
	Reps				
	Weight				
	Reps				
	Weight				
	Reps				
	Weight				
	Reps				
	Weight				
	Reps				
	Weight				
	Reps				

Mind Stuff

Thankful for

Future Perfect

Food and Drink Intake

Calories

Drinks

Supplements

Total

Mobility, Flexibility & Soft Tissue Work

Metabolic Disturbance

	fast (sec)	slow (secs)	no. of intervals
Unit of Resist.			

Strength Training

Exercise

	Weight				
	Reps				
	Weight				
	Reps				
	Weight				
	Reps				
	Weight				
	Reps				
	Weight				
	Reps				
	Weight				
	Reps				

Mind Stuff

Thankful for

Future Perfect

Food and Drink Intake

Calories

Drinks

Supplements

Total	

Mobility, Flexibility & Soft Tissue Work

Metabolic Disturbance

	fast (sec)	slow (secs)	no. of intervals
Unit of Resist.			

Strength Training

Exercise

	Weight				
	Reps				
	Weight				
	Reps				
	Weight				
	Reps				
	Weight				
	Reps				
	Weight				
	Reps				
	Weight				
	Reps				

Mind Stuff

Thankful for

Future Perfect

Food and Drink Intake

Calories

Drinks

Supplements

Total

Mobility, Flexibility & Soft Tissue Work

Metabolic Disturbance

	fast (sec)	slow (secs)	no. of intervals
Unit of Resist.			

Strength Training

Exercise

	Weight				
	Reps				
	Weight				
	Reps				
	Weight				
	Reps				
	Weight				
	Reps				
	Weight				
	Reps				
	Weight				
	Reps				

Mind Stuff

Thankful for

Future Perfect

Food and Drink Intake

Calories

Drinks

Supplements

Total

Mobility, Flexibility & Soft Tissue Work

Metabolic Disturbance

	fast (sec)	slow (secs)	no. of intervals
Unit of Resist.			

Strength Training

Exercise

Exercise					
	Weight				
	Reps				
	Weight				
	Reps				
	Weight				
	Reps				
	Weight				
	Reps				
	Weight				
	Reps				
	Weight				
	Reps				

Mind Stuff

Thankful for

Future Perfect

Food and Drink Intake

Calories

Drinks

Supplements

Total	

Mobility, Flexibility & Soft Tissue Work

Metabolic Disturbance

	fast (sec)	slow (secs)	no. of intervals

Unit of Resist.

Strength Training

Exercise

Exercise		Weight				
		Weight				
		Reps				
		Weight				
		Reps				
		Weight				
		Reps				
		Weight				
		Reps				
		Weight				
		Reps				
		Weight				
		Reps				

Mind Stuff

Thankful for

Future Perfect

Food and Drink Intake

Calories

Drinks

Supplements

Total	

Mobility, Flexibility & Soft Tissue Work

Metabolic Disturbance

	fast (sec)	slow (secs)	no. of intervals
Unit of Resist.			

Strength Training

Exercise

	Weight				
	Reps				
	Weight				
	Reps				
	Weight				
	Reps				
	Weight				
	Reps				
	Weight				
	Reps				
	Weight				
	Reps				

Mind Stuff

Thankful for

Future Perfect

Food and Drink Intake

Calories

Drinks

Supplements

Total

Mobility, Flexibility & Soft Tissue Work

Metabolic Disturbance

	fast (sec)	slow (secs)	no. of intervals
Unit of Resist.			

Strength Training

Exercise

	Weight				
	Reps				
	Weight				
	Reps				
	Weight				
	Reps				
	Weight				
	Reps				
	Weight				
	Reps				
	Weight				
	Reps				

Mind Stuff

Thankful for

Future Perfect

Food and Drink Intake

Calories

Drinks

Supplements

Total

Mobility, Flexibility & Soft Tissue Work

Metabolic Disturbance

	fast (sec)	slow (secs)	no. of intervals
Unit of Resist.			

Strength Training

Exercise

	Weight				
	Reps				
	Weight				
	Reps				
	Weight				
	Reps				
	Weight				
	Reps				
	Weight				
	Reps				
	Weight				
	Reps				

Mind Stuff

Thankful for

Future Perfect

Food and Drink Intake

Calories

Drinks

Supplements

Total

Mobility, Flexibility & Soft Tissue Work

Metabolic Disturbance

	fast (sec)	slow (secs)	no. of intervals
Unit of Resist.			

Strength Training

Exercise

	Weight				
	Reps				
	Weight				
	Reps				
	Weight				
	Reps				
	Weight				
	Reps				
	Weight				
	Reps				
	Weight				
	Reps				

Mind Stuff

Thankful for

Future Perfect

Food and Drink Intake

Calories

Drinks

Supplements

Total	

Mobility, Flexibility & Soft Tissue Work

Metabolic Disturbance

	fast (sec)	slow (secs)	no. of intervals
Unit of Resist.			

Strength Training

Exercise

	Weight				
	Reps				
	Weight				
	Reps				
	Weight				
	Reps				
	Weight				
	Reps				
	Weight				
	Reps				
	Weight				
	Reps				

Mind Stuff

Thankful for

Future Perfect

Food and Drink Intake

Calories

Drinks

Supplements

Total

Mobility, Flexibility & Soft Tissue Work

Metabolic Disturbance

	fast (sec)	slow (secs)	no. of intervals
Unit of Resist.			

Strength Training

Exercise

	Weight				
	Reps				
	Weight				
	Reps				
	Weight				
	Reps				
	Weight				
	Reps				
	Weight				
	Reps				
	Weight				
	Reps				

Mind Stuff

Thankful for

Future Perfect

Food and Drink Intake

Calories

Drinks

Supplements

Total

Mobility, Flexibility & Soft Tissue Work

Metabolic Disturbance

	fast (sec)	slow (secs)	no. of intervals
Unit of Resist.			

Strength Training

Exercise

	Weight				
	Reps				
	Weight				
	Reps				
	Weight				
	Reps				
	Weight				
	Reps				
	Weight				
	Reps				
	Weight				
	Reps				

Mind Stuff

Thankful for

Future Perfect

Food and Drink Intake

Calories

Drinks

Supplements

Total	

Mobility, Flexibility & Soft Tissue Work

Metabolic Disturbance

	fast (sec)	slow (secs)	no. of intervals
Unit of Resist.			

Strength Training

Exercise

	Weight				
	Reps				
	Weight				
	Reps				
	Weight				
	Reps				
	Weight				
	Reps				
	Weight				
	Reps				
	Weight				
	Reps				

Mind Stuff

Thankful for

Future Perfect

Food and Drink Intake

Calories

Drinks

Supplements

Total	

The McDonald's Diet Daily Training Record

Mobility, Flexibility & Soft Tissue Work

Metabolic Disturbance

	fast (sec)	slow (secs)	no. of intervals
Unit of Resist.			

Strength Training

Exercise

	Weight				
	Reps				
	Weight				
	Reps				
	Weight				
	Reps				
	Weight				
	Reps				
	Weight				
	Reps				
	Weight				
	Reps				

Mind Stuff

Thankful for

Future Perfect

Food and Drink Intake

Calories

Drinks

Supplements

Total

Mobility, Flexibility & Soft Tissue Work

Metabolic Disturbance

	fast (sec)	slow (secs)	no. of intervals
Unit of Resist.			

Strength Training

Exercise

Exercise					
	Weight				
	Reps				
	Weight				
	Reps				
	Weight				
	Reps				
	Weight				
	Reps				
	Weight				
	Reps				
	Weight				
	Reps				

Mind Stuff

Thankful for

Future Perfect

Food and Drink Intake

Calories

Drinks

Supplements

Total

Mobility, Flexibility & Soft Tissue Work

Metabolic Disturbance

	fast (sec)	slow (secs)	no. of intervals
Unit of Resist.			

Strength Training

Exercise

Exercise		Weight				
		Reps				
		Weight				
		Reps				
		Weight				
		Reps				
		Weight				
		Reps				
		Weight				
		Reps				
		Weight				
		Reps				

Mind Stuff

Thankful for

Future Perfect

Food and Drink Intake

	Calories

Drinks

Supplements

Total	

Mobility, Flexibility & Soft Tissue Work

Metabolic Disturbance

	fast (sec)	slow (secs)	no. of intervals

Unit of Resist.

Strength Training

Exercise

	Weight				
	Reps				
	Weight				
	Reps				
	Weight				
	Reps				
	Weight				
	Reps				
	Weight				
	Reps				
	Weight				
	Reps				

Mind Stuff

Thankful for

Future Perfect

Food and Drink Intake

	Calories

Drinks

Supplements

Total	

Mobility, Flexibility & Soft Tissue Work

Metabolic Disturbance

	fast (sec)	slow (secs)	no. of intervals

Unit of Resist.

Strength Training

Exercise

Exercise					
	Weight				
	Reps				
	Weight				
	Reps				
	Weight				
	Reps				
	Weight				
	Reps				
	Weight				
	Reps				
	Weight				
	Reps				

Mind Stuff

Thankful for

Future Perfect

Food and Drink Intake

	Calories

Drinks

Supplements

| Total | |

Mobility, Flexibility & Soft Tissue Work

Metabolic Disturbance

	fast (sec)	slow (secs)	no. of intervals
Unit of Resist.			

Strength Training

Exercise

	Weight				
	Reps				
	Weight				
	Reps				
	Weight				
	Reps				
	Weight				
	Reps				
	Weight				
	Reps				
	Weight				
	Reps				

Mind Stuff

Thankful for

Future Perfect

Food and Drink Intake

	Calories

Drinks

Supplements

Total	

Mobility, Flexibility & Soft Tissue Work

Metabolic Disturbance

	fast (sec)	slow (secs)	no. of intervals

Unit of Resist.

Strength Training

Exercise

	Weight				
	Reps				
	Weight				
	Reps				
	Weight				
	Reps				
	Weight				
	Reps				
	Weight				
	Reps				
	Weight				
	Reps				

Mind Stuff

Thankful for

Future Perfect

Food and Drink Intake

Calories

Drinks

Supplements

Total

Mobility, Flexibility & Soft Tissue Work

Metabolic Disturbance

	fast (sec)	slow (secs)	no. of intervals
Unit of Resist.			

Strength Training

Exercise

	Weight				
	Reps				
	Weight				
	Reps				
	Weight				
	Reps				
	Weight				
	Reps				
	Weight				
	Reps				
	Weight				
	Reps				

Mind Stuff

Thankful for

Future Perfect

Food and Drink Intake

Calories

Drinks

Supplements

Total	

Mobility, Flexibility & Soft Tissue Work

Metabolic Disturbance

	fast (sec)	slow (secs)	no. of intervals

Unit of Resist.

Strength Training

Exercise

	Weight				
	Reps				
	Weight				
	Reps				
	Weight				
	Reps				
	Weight				
	Reps				
	Weight				
	Reps				
	Weight				
	Reps				

Mind Stuff

Thankful for

Future Perfect

Food and Drink Intake

	Calories

Drinks

Supplements

Total	

Mobility, Flexibility & Soft Tissue Work

Metabolic Disturbance

	fast (sec)	slow (secs)	no. of intervals

Unit of Resist.

Strength Training

Exercise

Exercise					
	Weight				
	Reps				
	Weight				
	Reps				
	Weight				
	Reps				
	Weight				
	Reps				
	Weight				
	Reps				
	Weight				
	Reps				

Mind Stuff

Thankful for

Future Perfect

Food and Drink Intake

	Calories

Drinks

Supplements

Total	

Mobility, Flexibility & Soft Tissue Work

Metabolic Disturbance

	fast (sec)	slow (secs)	no. of intervals
Unit of Resist.			

Strength Training

Exercise

	Weight				
	Reps				
	Weight				
	Reps				
	Weight				
	Reps				
	Weight				
	Reps				
	Weight				
	Reps				
	Weight				
	Reps				

Mind Stuff

Thankful for

Future Perfect

Food and Drink Intake

Calories

Drinks

Supplements

Total	

Mobility, Flexibility & Soft Tissue Work

Metabolic Disturbance

	fast (sec)	slow (secs)	no. of intervals
Unit of Resist.			

Strength Training

Exercise

Weight				
Reps				
Weight				
Reps				
Weight				
Reps				
Weight				
Reps				
Weight				
Reps				
Weight				
Reps				

Mind Stuff

Thankful for

Future Perfect

Food and Drink Intake

	Calories

Drinks

Supplements

Total	

Mobility, Flexibility & Soft Tissue Work

Metabolic Disturbance

	fast (sec)	slow (secs)	no. of intervals
Unit of Resist.			

Strength Training

Exercise

	Weight			
	Reps			
	Weight			
	Reps			
	Weight			
	Reps			
	Weight			
	Reps			
	Weight			
	Reps			
	Weight			
	Reps			

Mind Stuff

Thankful for

Future Perfect

Food and Drink Intake

Calories

Drinks

Supplements

Total

Mobility, Flexibility & Soft Tissue Work

Metabolic Disturbance

	fast (sec)	slow (secs)	no. of intervals

Unit of Resist.

Strength Training

Exercise

	Weight				
	Reps				
	Weight				
	Reps				
	Weight				
	Reps				
	Weight				
	Reps				
	Weight				
	Reps				
	Weight				
	Reps				

Mind Stuff

Thankful for

Future Perfect

Food and Drink Intake

Calories

Drinks

Supplements

Total

Mobility, Flexibility & Soft Tissue Work

Metabolic Disturbance

	fast (sec)	slow (secs)	no. of intervals
Unit of Resist.			

Strength Training

Exercise

	Weight				
	Reps				
	Weight				
	Reps				
	Weight				
	Reps				
	Weight				
	Reps				
	Weight				
	Reps				
	Weight				
	Reps				

Mind Stuff

Thankful for

Future Perfect

Food and Drink Intake

Calories

Drinks

Supplements

Total	

Conclusion

The Diet

I would never recommend that anyone eat out every meal 7 days a week, no matter where. The majority of your meals should be made from fresh, natural ingredients, cooked and eaten at home.

Having said that, if you are looking for a delicious, healthy, and super convenient meal that is low in calories, carbohydrates and fat and high in protein (29g per serving) you would have to go a long way to beat the McDonald's Grilled Chicken Caesar Salad with Balsamic Dressing.

If you rush to work without having time to prepare a lunch to take with you and end up choosing the best from a bad selection from the company canteen or the nearest deli or fast food joint, then you no longer have any excuse. McDonald's are everywhere, and the Chicken Salad which packs only 210 Calories, including the Balsamic Dressing is the perfect choice.

If you buy takeaways or frozen meals on your way home at night to save cooking dinner, same thing. If it is not filling enough for you as a dinner, add a couple of cups of fresh, raw baby spinach or lightly steamed broccoli or asparagus (or all three) and mix it all up in a bowl with the Balsamic Dressing and you have a very satisfying meal, loaded with nutrition, yet low in calories.

For the purposes of this experiment I didn't add anything, but in future I certainly will. I ate almost one hundred of these salads in 30 days, and I never tired of them. So if you can pimp them out with different green veggies, you shouldn't either. I kept all my receipts over the month and I ended up buying a lot more than 100 salads because my wife chose to eat one or two every day, even though she could have eaten whatever she wanted.

If you plan to follow my journey to weight loss I would recommend that you substitute at least some of the salads with steamed green vegetables and a piece of grilled, low fat beef, chicken, turkey or fish.

And at just 45 calories per portion, the Fruit Bags are an excellent snack. Between dinner and bedtime is often a dangerous time for eating. Your body does not need any additional calories but you feel peckish, so out come the biscuits, potato crisps or chocolates. A normal portion of any of those will add around 500 calories to your day.

They are also great for the movies. I would eat 1 or 2 bags plus a bottle of mineral water, for a total of 90 calories. The people sitting around me with the popcorn, candy and sodas were getting in 600 to 1,000, depending the sizes.

You could definitely prepare your own fruits cheaper, but will you? I found the convenience made it just so easy to do. I always kept a good supply in my refrigerator at home, and the rest of my family ate more fruit during that month than they have ever eaten before.

In fact one of the big reasons for the success of this diet is its convenience and simplicity. Unlike most diets, with McDonald's there are no grey areas. The salads, Fruit Bags and water are good all day long. The burgers and wraps only straight after a workout. The fries and desserts should be only be eaten once you have reached your goal weight, and then only occasionally.

The Training

Under normal circumstances I would not change my exercise selection around so quickly. I would usually use the same exercises for about 6 weeks, only increasing the weight whenever I could.

The exception would be if you are using a regression. In that case as soon as you could do the base exercise, you should. For example if you cannot do full body weight squats you would start out squatting to a chair. If after 2 weeks you realized you could now do full squats, you would immediately switch to those.

The reason I changed so often was to show you a lot of different exercises and how they would fit into the program.

I would change the rep ranges every 2 weeks. So the first 2 weeks I would use a weight with which I could do 15 reps. The next 2 weeks a weight for 12 reps and the following 2 weeks 8 reps. Obviously as the reps come down the weight would be increasing.

I would then change the exercises and go back to 15 reps, and so on.

We are all different, and even if you follow my eating and training plan exactly, the results will not be identical. Some of you will lose a little less weight, most of you will probably lose more. This is because my starting weight was not that far from my goal weight. The last 10 pounds are always the hardest to lose. Most of my weight loss was those last 10 pounds.

If you have any questions please have a look at the FAQ under the McDonald's Diet tab on my website. If your question is not answered, then post it and look back awhile later.

It has been an interesting journey, I am in the best shape of my life, I feel great, and life is good. In fact . . . I'm lovin' it !

```
*************************************
```

B+H. Zobrist
McDonald's Restaurant
Adlikerstrasse 297
8105 Regensdorf
Tel: 044 870 01 05
Fax:044 870 01 06

```
*************************************
```

Vielen Dank für Ihren Besuch

```
*************************************
```

QUITTUNG

No TVA: MWST NR 265 914#ORD 59
01/05/2010 19:03:44
ANZ PROD
  5 CA-GRILLED
  10 BALSAMICO
  5 FRUIT BAG

Take-Out Total
CHF
Change

TAX B (2.40%)   59.
***   Öffnungszei
Sonntag - Donnerstag
Freitag und Samstag

MCDONALD'S Restaurant
NIEDERHASLISTRASSE 7
8157 DIELSDORF
Tel 044 854 06 09
Hern Beat Zobrist

```
*************************************
```

Vielen Dank für Ihren Besuch
McDonald's wünscht Ihnen einen
excellenten Appetit

```
*************************************
```

QUITTUNG

No TVA: MWST NR 265 914#ORD 49 -REG
22/04/2010 13:29:57
ANZ PROD
  1 SMAL VALSER   TOTAL
  1 McCHIKEN   3.50
                                 6.10
Take-Out Total
CHF   9.60
Change   10.60
                                1.00
TAX B (2.40%)
                    9.60 =   0.23
***   Oeffnungszeiten   ***
Montag - Donnerstag : 08h30 - 23h30
Freitag und Samstag : 08h30 - 01h00
Sonntag   : 10h30 - 23h30
```
```

Glossary

Abdominals: The muscles in front of the abdomen (stomach area). They support the spine when lifting things or making big movements. They transfer power from the legs to the upper body. They are often abbreviated to the "abs" and include the muscles making up the "six pack"

BMR: The rate at which your body burns calories at rest to maintain normal body functions. It is the amount of calories you burn per day, excluding exercise. It differs from person to person based on age, weight, height, gender, diet and exercise habits.

Barbell: A long metal bar (4 to 7 feet) to which weight discs are attached at each end.

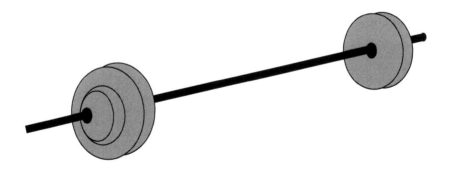

Dumbbell: A short bar (around 1 foot) with metal balls or weight discs attached to each end. Usually used in pairs.

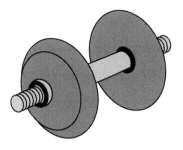

Good Exercise Form: To perform an exercise as it should be done. This includes correct tempo (exercise speed), range of movement and only moving the body parts that should move.

Grips:

  Neutral Grip: A grip in which your palms face each other

  Pronated Grip: A grip in which your palms face down

  Supinated Grip: A grip in which your palms face up

Kettle bell: A traditional Russian cast iron weight looking somewhat like a cannonball with a handle.

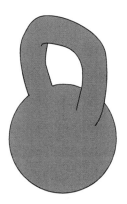

Lats: The large muscles situated on the back of the trunk and to the sides. They give lean, well developed men the "V-shape"

Rep Ranges: The number of repetitions you do within a certain range will have different results. For example if you do sets of between 1 and 5 repetitions, the main effect of this will be to increase strength. 6 - 12 reps is for building muscle and over 15 would be for muscle endurance. There is overlap in all rep ranges, in other words if you steadily increased the amount of weight you could lift for 15 reps, your strength would also increase. But the primary effect in this case would be an increase in muscle endurance.

Repetition: The most basic element of a workout. Performing an exercise once, for example lifting and then lowering a weight once is one repetion. (usually abbreviated to one rep or several reps)

Resistance: Anything which increases the force required to perform a movement. This could simply mean more weight on a barbell or machine, or a heavier dumbbell. Resistance can also be in the form of your own body weight. Changing your body position in certain exercises will increase or decrease the resistance.

Rest Period: The amount of time taken to recover between sets. For weight loss and muscle building 30 - 60 seconds is best. For strength, somewhat longer.

Set: A set is a group of repetitions. For example if you had to do 3 sets of 12 reps (abbreviated as 3 x 12) you would complete 12 repetitions and then either take a break or do something else and then start over, do something else, and then do your last set of 12 reps.

About the Author

Mark Austin is a Certified Personal Trainer and a Certified Specialist in Performance Nutrition.

He has been in the fitness industry since 1985.

During the 90's he founded and co-owned the biggest chain of fitness clubs in the Southern Hemisphere and co-founded and co-owned the biggest gym equipment manufacturing company in South Africa.

During this time he had over 1,000 workouts with Arnold Schwarzenegger's mentor, Reg Park.

Currently he owns Austin Fitness, a personal training business in Switzerland specializing in rapid weight loss.

References

Disclaimer and Caution

1 Dr. Stuart McGill - *"Ultimate Back Fitness and Performance"*

The Results

1 American Council on Exercise

2 American Heart Association

3 American Heart Association

4 Dr. Melissa Palmer's - *"Guide of Hepatitis and Liver Disease"*

Supplementation

1 American Institute for Cancer Research

2 The American Heart Association

3 Harvard School of Public Health

4 The Royal Adelaide Hospital

5 Professor Peter Howe of the University of South Australia

6 Fern et al. and Meredith et al.

The Diet

1 Abate M, Di Iorio A, Di Renzo D, Paganelli R, Saggini R, Abate G (September 2007). *"Frailty in the elderly: the physical dimension"*

2 Dr. Donald Layman, professor of food science and human nutrition at the University of Illinois

3 Dr. William Berkowitz - *"The Experts Guide to Weight Loss"*

4 Alwyn Cosgrove - *"Afterburn"*

5 Joel Marion - *"Cheat Your Way Thin"*

Exercise

1 Dr. Lawrence Morehouse – Author of the sections on exercise and physiology for the *Encyclopedia Americana, the Encyclopedia Britannica and the Encyclopedia of Sports Medicine.*

2 Dr. Dicken Weatherby - *"Naturally Raising your HGH Levels"*

3 Rachel Cosgrove - *"The Female Body Breakthrough"*

4 Eric Cressey - *"Maximum Strength"*

Psychology of Weight Loss

1 The Cleveland Clinic

2 R. Emmons and M. McCullough - *"The Psychology of Gratitude"*

3 Burton, C. M., & King, L. A. (2009). *"The Benefits of Writing About PositiveExperiences"*